Community Health Nursing
RECORD BOOK
for PB BSc Nursing Program

Community Health Nursing RECORD BOOK

for PB BSc Nursing Program

C Manivannan MSc (N) MSc (Psy) MPhil (Psy) CMLT
Principal
Norang Ram Dayanand Dhukia Nursing College
Jhunjhunu, Rajasthan, India

T Latha Manivannan MSc (N)
Assistant Professor
Department of Community Health Nursing
Norang Ram Dayanand Dhukia Nursing College
Jhunjhunu, Rajasthan, India

S Rathamani MSc (N)
Vice Principal and Head
Department of Community Health Nursing
Sri Vishnu Nursing College
Bengaluru, Karnataka, India

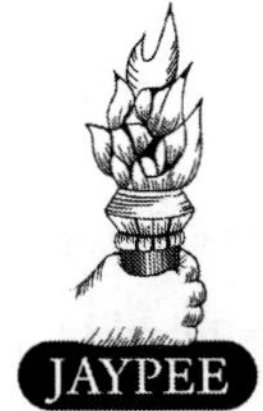

JAYPEE BROTHERS MEDICAL PUBLISHERS
The Health Sciences Publisher
New Delhi | London

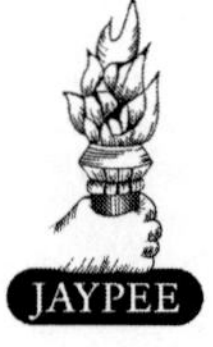

Jaypee Brothers Medical Publishers (P) Ltd

Headquarters
EMCA House
23/23-B, Ansari Road, Daryaganj
New Delhi - 110 002, India
Landline: +91-11-23272143, +91-11-23272703
+91-11-23282021, +91-11-23245672
E-mail: jaypee@jaypeebrothers.com

Corporate Office
4838/24, Ansari Road, Daryaganj
New Delhi - 110 002, India
Phone: +91-11-43574357
Fax: +91-11-43574314
E-mail: jaypee@jaypeebrothers.com

Overseas Office
J.P. Medical Ltd
83 Victoria Street, London
SW1H 0HW (UK)
Phone: +44 20 3170 8910
E-mail: info@jpmedpub.com

EU GPSR Authorised Representative
Logos Europe, 9 rue Nicolas Poussin
17000, La Rochelle, France
Phone: +33 (0) 6 67 93 73 78
E-mail: contact@logoseurope.eu

Website: www.jaypeebrothers.com
Website: www.jaypeedigital.com

Inquiries for bulk sales may be solicited at: jaypee@jaypeebrothers.com

Community Health Nursing Record Book for PB BSc Nursing Program

First Edition: 2016

Reprint: **2026**

ISBN 978-93-5250-134-2

Printed at: *Samrat Offset Pvt. Ltd.*

Dedicated to

Our parents
Chinnusamy and Muthulakshmi
Thangavel and Angammal
Subramani and Thulasimani
and
All students of nursing profession

PREFACE

Community Health Nursing Record Book for PB BSc Nursing Program is prepared according to the requirements of community health nursing for PB BSc nursing course. It provides simple and systematic record book on this field for undergraduate students. The PB BSc Nursing students guided by their teachers in various aspects are expected to maintain quality and standard for community experience based on requirements, which were established for every college of nursing.

This record book is updated and is based on Indian Nursing Council (INC) syllabus, which is specially organized for PB BSc Nursing Program in Community Health Nursing for second year students. This record book has portrayed the subject in 23 procedures with important notes and explanations, which would definitely meet the demands of students.

This book helps maintain good community experience based on requirements with standardized format, which minimize the workload of clinical instructor and students. The students would be self-guided by this book at the time of community visit. These formats are standardized and based on community requirements that can be followed by the students easily. It also helps the students maintain all the records of community experience, which would help the clinical instructor evaluate the student's activity in the community area.

We hope that this book would be an asset in the field of Community Health Nursing.

C Manivannan
T Latha Manivannan
S Rathamani

ACKNOWLEDGMENTS

First of all, we would like to thank Almighty for giving us strength, patience and good health to complete this book successfully.

We owe our heartiest and greatest thanks to Chairman, Rukmini Shetty Memorial College of Nursing and Sri Venkateshwara College of Nursing, Bengaluru, Karnataka, India, for constant encouragement and support.

We express our warm gratitude to all our colleagues and friends for their constant encouragement for writing this record book. We take this opportunity to express our sincere thanks to our parents, sisters and brothers for their unselfish love, endless patience and quite understanding that allowed us to complete this book successfully.

Last but not least, we express our warm gratitude to Shri Jitendar P Vij (Group Chairman), Mr Ankit Vij (Group President), Mr Tarun Duneja (Director-Publishing) and all staff of Bengaluru branch, especially Mr Kumar C, Sales Executive of M/s Jaypee Brothers Medical Publishers (P) Ltd, New Delhi, India, for their constant encouragement for publishing this book.

STUDENT'S PROFILE

Name of the Institution : ________________________
(IN BLOCK LETTERS)
Place : ________________________
Name of the Student : ________________________
Register Number : ________________________
Date of Posting : From: __________ To: __________
Month and Year of Joining : ________________________
Signature of the Student : ________________________

PHOTOGRAPH

Name and Signature of Clinical Instructor
Date:

Name and Signature
Head of Department of Community Health Nursing
Date:

Name and Signature of Principal
Date:

College Seal

Name and Signature of Internal Examiner
Date:

1.
2.

Name and Signature of External Examiner
Date:

1.
2.

CONTENTS

ESSENTIAL REQUIREMENTS OF COMMUNITY HEALTH NURSING FOR POST BASIC BSc NURSING PROGRAM

Sl No.	Requirements	No. of requirements	Date of completion of requirements
1.	Orientation Report	1	
2.	Primary Health Center Report	1	
3.	Community Survey	1	
4.	Household Survey	5	
5.	Family Folder	5	
6.	Family Care Plan	3	
7.	Family Care Study	2	
8.	Antenatal Clinic	1	
9.	Postnatal Clinic	1	
10.	Under-five Clinic	1	
11.	Family Welfare Clinic	1	
12.	Antenatal Assessment	5	
13	Postnatal Assessment	5	
14.	Preschool Assessment	3	
15.	Newborn Assessment	3	
16.	Old Age Assessment	3	
17.	Nutritional Assessment of Under-five Children	5	
18.	Cooking Demonstration	2	
19.	Observation Visit	4	
20.	Bag Technique Procedure		
	• Temperature Taking	2	
	• Urine Test	2	
	• Dressing	2	
	• Oral Medication	5	
	• Injection	2	
21.	Health Education	2	
22.	Audiovisual Aids Preparation	7	
23.	Organization of Health Camp	1	

Signature of Student
Date:

Signature of Clinical Instructor
Date:

Signature of Head of Department of Community Health Nursing
Date:

Signature of Principal

Date:

General Objectives of Community Visit

Purpose of the Experience

- The students understand the administrative setup and functions of administration in different areas of nursing service that is in the community health nursing setup.
- They are able to identify and analyze the problem in administration and suggest possible remedies with the application of problem solving.
- The students are able to identify and critically analyze the existing problems in administration.

Requirements for Short Notes on Community Health Nursing During Practice

Community Health Nursing

A field of nursing that is a blend of primary health care and nursing practice with public health nursing. The community health nurse conducts a continuing and comprehensive practice, i.e. preventive, curative and rehabilitative. The philosophy of care is based on the belief that care directed to the individual, family, and group contributes to the health care of the population as a whole. The community health nurse is not restricted to the care of a particular age or diagnostic group. Participation of all consumers of health care is encouraged in the development of community activities that contribute to the promotion of education and maintenance of good health. These activities require comprehensive health program that pay special attention to social and ecologic influences, and specific populations at risk.

PURPOSE OF THE EXPERIENCE

The students understand the administrative setup and functions of administration in different areas of nursing service that is in the community health setup and are able to identify, and analyze the problem in administration and suggest possible remedies with the application of problem solving. The students are able to identify and critically analyze the existing problem in administration.

METHODS OF STUDY

1. Observation.
2. Questionnaire.
3. Discussion with concerned personnel in each area.
4. Written assignments.
5. Presentation of reports:
   a. Describe the community health nursing setup as you observed.
   b. Students are able to understand and explain:
      - Community health nursing administration organized on healthcare delivery system, 5 year plan and primary health care
      - Scope of community health nursing (administrative supervisory teaching and research)
      - Functions of public health nurse in homes, clinic, urban, rural, general and special
      - Health centers: Rural primary health centers, subcenters and urban primary health centers
      - Hospitals and industries
      - Training at community health centers, teaching institutions, schools and colleges of nursing, and multipurpose worker's school
      - Regional family welfare training center
      - Institute of public health
      - District public health office: General and family welfare
      - Health education bureau: Central and state
      - Applied nutrition program
      - National welfare, control and eradication programs for tuberculosis, leprosy, malaria and others

- Special projects, World Health Organization (WHO), Danish International Development Agency (DANIDA) and homes for handicapped children and others
- Responsibilities of community health nurse in the care of handicapped children
- Implication of the aging population in relation to preventive and social medicine problems
- Community health program planning steps:
  - Plan formation
  - Execution
  - Evaluation
  - Health needs and demands
  - Resources
  - Objectives
  - Targets
  - Goals
  - Plans.
- Community organization
- Role of community leaders:
  - Identification and training of community leaders
  - Training and supervision of community level workers.

TERMINOLOGY

- Infection:
  - The entry and development or multiplication of disease producing agent in the body of man or animal may or may not lead to disease.
- Epidemic:
  - An outbreak of disease in a community in excess of normal expectation and derived from a common source (e.g. cholera).
- Endemic:
  - The condition, which is present within the population.
- Sporadic:
  - The incidence at intervals of single scattered cares of disease.
- Pandemic:
  - An epidemic, which is spreads from country to country or whole world.
- Zoonosis:
  - Disease, which is transmitted from animal to man.
- Communicable disease:
  - An illness due to specific infectious agent, which is spread from one person to another person.
- Non-communicable disease:
  - Which is applied in case of anemia and diabetes mellitus.
- Incubation period:
  - This is the time interval between entry of disease agent into the body and its appearing of the first signs and symptoms.
- Isolation:
  - Separation of patient with infectious disease.
- Antiserum:
  - Serum contain specific antibody.
- Carrier:
  - A person who carries the disease agent.

- Fomites:
  - In animate article other than food and water. For example, pen, pencil and handkerchief.
- Vector:
  - Usually an anthropoid, which transfer infection to person.
- Virulent:
  - Measuring the severity of diseases.
- Pathogenesis:
  - Ability to cause disease.
- Agent:
  - A biological, physical, chemical entry capable of causing diseases.
- Antibody:
  - A protein substance producing resistance, power, naturally or artificially.
- Antigen:
  - It is a foreign body.
- Attack rate:
  - A measurement of the frequency of new cases.

PRINCIPLES OF COMMUNITY HEALTH NURSING

1. Community health nurse provide care based on needs of individuals, families and communities.
2. The community health nurse has to achieve the goal use of knowledge and understanding the objectives, and policies of the agency.
3. Community health nurse considers the family is the fundamental unit for providing preventive, promotive and curative services.
4. Respect the values, customs and beliefs of the clients contribute to the effectiveness of care to the client. Community health nurse service must be available sustainable and affordable to all regardless of race, creed, color and socioeconomic status.
5. Community health nurse integrated health education and counseling as vital parts of functions. They encourage and support community peoples to improve the health.
6. Community health nurse has to improve relationships with the co-workers and members of the health team facilities accomplishments of goals. Each member is helped to see how his/her work benefits the whole enterprise.
7. Community health nurse should have periodic and continuing evaluation work to fulfill and achieve goals, and objectives of program. Clients are involved in the appraisal of their health program through consultations, observations and accurate recording.
8. Community health nurses should have professional interest; they consider formulating plan of staff development programs to improve the quality service. It is essential to upgrade and maintain sound nursing practices.
9. Utilization of indigenous and existing community resources, there by maximizing the success of the efforts of the community health nurses. The use of local available ailments, linkages with existing community resources, both public and private, increase the awareness of what care they need and what are entitled?
10. Community health nursing program need active participation of the individual, family and community in planning, and making decisions for their healthcare needs, determine, to a large extent, then it will successes. Organized community groups are encouraged to participate in the activities that will meet community needs and interests.
11. Supervision of nursing services by qualified community health nursing personnel to provide guidance and direction to the work to be done. Potentials of employees for effective and efficient work are developed.

12. Accurate recording and reporting serve as the basis for evaluation of the progress of planned programs and activities, and as a guide for the future actions. Maintenance of accurate records one vital responsibility of community as these are utilized in studies and researches and as legal documents.

LEVELS OF PREVENTION

The goals of medicine are to promote health, preventive disease and restore health, when it is impaired. The levels are primordial prevention, primary prevention, secondary prevention and tertiary prevention.

Primordial Prevention

1. It is a new concept, is receiving special attention in the prevention of chronic disease it is the purest form of primary prevention that is prevention of risk factors, e.g. obesity, hypertension. Good lifestyles can prevent the disease, e.g. exercise. Bad habits are harmful to health, e.g. smoking.
2. Efforts are directed towards discouraging children from adoptive harmful lifestyle.
3. Health education will provide intervention for individual to prevent the disease.

Primary Prevention

1. Action taken prior to the onset of disease, which removes the possibility that a disease will ever occur.
2. It significance intervention in the prepathogenesis phase.
3. It includes the concept of positive health, a concept that encourages achievement and maintenance of an acceptable level of health that will enable every individual to lead socially and economically protective life.
4. The concept of primary prevention is now being apply to the prevention of chronic disease such as coronary heart disease, hypertension and cancer based on elimination or modification of risk factors of disease.

Secondary Prevention

It can be defined as actions taken, which halt's the progress of a disease at its incipient stage and prevent complication.

Intervention

1. Early diagnosis and adequate treatment (screening test).
2. By early diagnosis and treatment, secondary prevention attempt to arrest the disease process, restore health by seeking out unrecognized disease treating it before irreversible pathological changes, now taken place and reverse communicability infectious disease.
3. It protect others in the community from the infection.
4. They provide secondary prevention for the infected individuals and primary prevention for their contacts.
5. It is largely the domain of clinical medicine.
6. The health programs initiated by governments, usually at the level of secondary prevention.
7. The drawback of secondary prevention is that the patient has already been subject to mental anguish, physical and the community to lose a production.
8. It is an imperfective tool in the control of transmission of disease.
9. It is more expensive and less effective.

Tertiary Prevention

1. When the disease process has advantage beyond its easy stages.
2. It is still possible to accomplish prevention by what might be call tertiary prevention.

3. Its significance is intervention in the late pathogenesis phase.
4. Tertiary prevention can be defined as all measure available to reduce all limit impairment and disability, minimize suffering caused by existence departure from good health and promote the patient adjustment to immediate condition. For example, treatment even in undertake late in the natural history of disease may prevent sequence and limit disability.
5. When defect and disability have more or less stabilized producer and its own pattern of disease?
6. The term of this will be obvious, when on compares the leading causes of death in developed countries.

PROCEDURES DURING HOME VISIT

Bag Technique

1. The community bag consists of front pouch, side pouches, lower compartment and upper compartment. Front pouch consist of hand washing articles such as soap with soap dish, nail brush, nail cutter and towel.
2. The front side pouch consists of newspaper and physical examination articles such as scale, fetus scope, stethoscope, inch tape, etc.
3. The backside pouch consists of paper bag, hemoglobin estimation scale, pen, paper, diary, etc.
4. The lower compartment consists of clean articles such as kidney tray, spirit lamp, test tube holder, match box, etc.
5. The upper compartment consist of sterile articles such as temperature pack, dressing pack, injection pack, oral medications, injections, solutions, ointment, test tube, slides, etc.:
   a. Always keep the bag at the right side.
   b. Take the newspaper and spread the newspaper, the inner side should be in up.
   c. Keep the bag at the corner of the newspaper and the front pouch should be placed at the backside.
   d. First take the handwashing articles from the front pouch.
   e. Take the needed articles from the clean compartment or side pouches.
   f. Do handwashing.
   g. Take the needed articles from the upper compartment.
   h. Close the upper compartment.
   i. Do the procedure.
   j. Clean the articles.
   k. Do handwashing.
   l. Replace the sterile articles first and replace the clean articles, and side pouch articles.
   m. Replace the handwashing articles.
   n. Close the bag.

Temperature Technique

1. Open the front pouch takes the handwashing articles.
2. Open the side pouch takes the paper bag diary and pen.
3. Open the lower compartment takes the kidney tray.
4. Do handwashing.
5. Open the sterile compartment and take the temperature pack. It consists of thermometer, cotton balls and cotton pad.
6. Close the upper compartment.
7. Open the thermometer pack, take the thermometer from the pouch, take one cotton ball and clean the thermometer from bulb to stem, and discard in the paper bag.
8. Keep the thermometer under the tongue of the client.

9. Wait for 3 minutes, remove the thermometer, take another cotton ball to clean from stem to bulb and discard in the paper bag.
10. Read the mercury level and record in the diary.
11. Take the cotton pad, wet it and applies the soap and rolls the thermometer, and keep it in the kidney tray for 3 minutes.
12. After 3 minutes remove the soapy cotton to discard in the paper bag.
13. Wash the thermometer under the running water.
14. Take another cotton ball, clean the thermometer stem to bulb and keep it in the pouch.
15. Burn the paper bag.
16. Clean the kidney tray.
17. Do handwashing.
18. Replace the thermometer pouch in the upper compartment.
19. Replace the kidney tray in the lower compartment.
20. Replace the handwashing articles and close the bag.

Urine Test

1. Open the bag, takes the handwashing articles.
2. Open the side pouch to take pen and diary.
3. Open the lower compartment, take the kidney tray, specimen bottle, spirit lamp, match box and test tube holder.
4. Do handwashing.
5. Open the upper compartment, take test tubes and solutions.
6. Close the bag.
7. Take the test tube, hold it in test tube holder, pour 5 mL of Benedict's solution and heat it.
8. Watch the color change, if it is blue continue or if any color change discard it.
9. In 5 mL of Benedict's solution, after the heating add eight drops of urine and boil it.
10. Make it, cool and watch the color change:
    - Blue : Negative
    - Green : 1%
    - Yellow : 2%
    - Orange : 3%
    - Brick red : Above 5%.
11. Enter the result.
12. Discard the waste.
13. Clean the articles.
14. Do handwashing.
15. Replace the upper compartment articles and replace the lower compartment articles.
16. Replace the handwashing articles.
17. Close the bag.

Dressing

1. Open the bag, take the handwashing articles.
2. Open the side pouch, take paper bag, diary and pen.
3. Open the lower compartment, take the kidney tray.
4. Remove the old dressing and discard in the kidney tray.
5. Do handwashing.

6. Open the upper compartment, take the dressing pack consists of artery forceps, thumb forceps, scissor, cotton balls, gauze piece, needed ointment and solutions.
7. Open the dressing pack, take artery forceps take one cotton dip it in the normal saline clean the wound from center to periphery.
8. Take another cotton dip it in the solution and squeeze it in the kidney tray, and clean the wound from center to periphery.
9. Take the ointment; apply over the wound with the help of cotton.
10. Keep the cotton pack covered with gauze to prevent from sticking the wound.
11. Tie with gauze or put the plaster.
12. Clean all the articles if facility available boil the water and put the instruments inside the water for 10–15 minutes.
13. If facility is not available take one plastic cover put the used articles inside and sterilize in health center.
14. Do handwashing.
15. Replace the upper compartment articles.
16. Replace lower compartment articles.
17. Replace the handwashing articles.
18. Record the procedure.

Oral Medication

1. Open the front pouch and take the handwashing articles.
2. Open the side pouch and take paper bag.
3. Do handwashing.
4. Open the upper compartment and take the needed medication.
5. Get the water from the client home and ask the client to open the mouth and swallow the medication with water. Observe that if the client swallowed the medication or not especially in under-fives.
6. Discard the waste in the paper bag and burn the paper bag.
7. Do the handwashing.
8. Replace the handwashing articles.
9. Close the bag.
10. Record the procedure with medicine name, dose, route and action.

Intramuscular Injection (If Standing Order Permitted)

1. Open the bag and take the handwashing articles.
2. Open the side pouch take pen, diary and paper bag.
3. Do handwashing.
4. Open the upper compartment and take the injection pack consists of syringe, needle, dry cotton, ampule cutter, also take spirit and needed medication.
5. Open the pack, take the syringe and needle, cut the ampule with the help of ampule cutter if it is the vial, open the vial and take the medicine.
6. Select the site clean with spirit cotton and administer injection intramuscularly.
7. Remove the syringe and needle, and massage the site.
8. Discard the waste in the paper bag and burn the paper bag.
9. Clean the articles.
10. Do handwashing.
11. Replace the articles.
12. Record the procedure.

Cord Care

Prevention of infection is very important as the newborns are not only susceptible by succumb quickly to infections. The risks are higher in low-birth-weight babies, especially preterm.

Purpose

1. To prevent infection.
2. To promote healing power.
3. To clean the cord.

Procedure

1. Take handwashing articles from the bag.
2. Get the paper bag ready.
3. Wash hands thoroughly with soap and water.
4. Allow your hands to dry in the air.
5. Inform the mother.
6. Take out the items needed from sterile compartment.
7. Spread out the central hole towel on the abdomen. Only the cord or umbilicus should be exposed.
8. Keeps small tray containing forceps on the towel.
9. Take the artery forceps and use cotton balls inside the pack.
10. Pour the antiseptic in a small bowl.
11. Clean the cord from central to the periphery.
12. Discard the cotton swab in a paper bag.
13. Repeat the procedure until it is cleaned.
14. Dispose the used swabs by burning or burial.
15. Need not apply any medicine expect spirit or Betadine.
16. Do not cover the umbilical cord and leave it open.
17. Wash the items and boil the tray with instruments in the home itself for next use.
18. Wash the hands with soap and water.
19. Replace the articles inside the bag.
20. Give necessary instruction.
21. Plan for next visit.
22. Record the procedure and observations made.

Diabetic Foot Care Procedures

The highest incidents of non-traumatic lower leg amputation involve diabetic patients, according to Medical News Today. Nerve damage and poor blood flow causes small injuries to quickly escalate, however, amputation is preventable with proper foot care. Keeping a diabetics' foot healthy is critical and foot care procedures take only a small amount of time a day.

Inspection

Daily visual foot inspections are recommended. A person with poor eyesight should ask for assistance with foot inspections. Patients should look and feel for any signs of injury. A diabetic patient must understand even a small cut or bruise quickly turns into an infected area, if left untreated. Signs of possible foot problems include redness, swelling, foot odor, bruising and loss of hair on toes. Occasionally, a diabetic's foot fractures, yet the patient remain unaware of the injury because of decreased circulation and sensory loss.

Diabetics may even walk on the fractured foot for several days to weeks without realizing that the foot has become severely injured. Major deformities and further complications may occur. Signs of a foot fracture include redness, increased temperature and change in form or shape. Also, immediate medical attention is required.

Wash Feet

Wash feet daily with warm water and soap. A diabetic should test water with his/her hand or wrist prior to placing feet into it. A diabetic's foot may not feel extreme heat and burn injuries could occur. Rubbing a pumice stone on hard areas of the foot removes the formation of corns and calluses. A person should polish the stone on wet feet. Never attempt cutting calluses off or use chemicals, advises the Diabetes Foundation. Drying feet thoroughly is important to removing water buildup.

Moisturize

Moisturizing the skin after bathing is critical. A diabetic patient's foot no longer emits oils, which leads to cracking and extreme dryness, explains the Diabetes Association. The association recommends applying a thin layer of petroleum jelly or other non-fragrance ointment to the foot. A person with diabetes should not apply the lotion between the toes where increased moisture leads to bacterial and fungal growth, which are difficult to heal in a diabetic condition.

Footwear

Diabetics are discouraged to walk around barefoot due to the increased risk of injury. Soft, seamless socks are encouraged as well as wearing house shoes indoors. Diabetics should always feel inside a shoe for loose pebbles or other items before putting a shoe on. The Diabetes Association explain nerves in the foot may have become unable to detect something inside the shoe. Shoes should fit comfortably with enough room around the sides and toes to prevent squeezing from occurring. Special shoes made for diabetics are available and often covered by insurance plans.

Health Education

Health education is an essential tool of communication in community health. It has been integrated in all the functions of primary health center.

Purpose

1. To motivate people and help them.
2. Maintain and adopt health practices in their daily life.
3. To bring out the behavioral changes.
4. To include the habits of personal hygiene.

Steps

1. Selection of topic according to the felt needs of the people.
2. Get ready with the articles or necessary audiovisual (AV) aids.
3. Inform your group and motivate them.
4. Speak in an informal way.
5. Select the teaching aids and start with known to unknown.
6. Speak with them in their own language.
7. Select the work area and fix the charts or posters that should be visible to everyone.

8. Use appropriate diagram in the flash card.
9. Use always pointer.
10. Hold the flash cards below the chest level.
11. Explain the story in a narrative from without seeing the cards.
12. Flow of speech should not be disturbed.
13. Make them understand well.
14. Rotate only your body and do not to move here and there.
15. Flash cards should be 12–16 in numbers.
16. Follow the principles of AV aids.
17. Encourage participation.
18. Ask questions during health teaching program.

THEORIES APPLIED IN COMMUNITY HEALTH NURSING

The concept of community is defined as "a group of people who share some important feature of their lives and use some common agencies, and institutions." The concept of health is defined as "a balanced state of well-being resulting from harmonious interactions of body, mind and spirit." The term community health is defined by meeting the needs of a community by identifying problems and managing interactions within the community.

Basic Elements

The six basic elements of nursing practice incorporated in community health programs and services are:

1. Promotion of healthful living.
2. Prevention of health problems.
3. Treatment of disorders.
4. Rehabilitation.
5. Evaluation.
6. Research.

Major Roles

The focus of nursing includes not only the individual but also the family and the community, meeting these multiple needs requires multiple roles. The seven major roles of a community health nurse are:

1. Care provider.
2. Educator.
3. Advocate.
4. Manager.
5. Collaborator.
6. Leader.
7. Researcher.

Major Settings

Settings for community health nursing can be grouped into six categories:

1. Homes.
2. Ambulatory care settings.
3. Schools.
4. Occupational health settings.

5. Residential institutions.
6. The community at large.

Community health nursing practice is not limited to a specific area, but can be practiced anywhere.

THEORIES AND MODELS FOR COMMUNITY HEALTH NURSING

The commonly used theories are:

1. Nightingale's theory of environment.
2. Orem's self-care model.
3. Neuman's healthcare system model.
4. Roger's model of the science and unitary man.
5. Pender's health promotion model.
6. Roy's adaptation model.
7. Milio's framework of prevention.
8. Salmon White's construct for public health nursing.
9. Block and Josten's ethical theory of population focused nursing.
10. Canadian model.
11. Kurt Lewin's theory of social changes.

Milio's Framework of Prevention

1. Nancy Milio is a nurse and leader in public health policy, and public health education developed a framework for prevention that includes concepts of community-oriented and population focused care (1976, 1981).
2. The basic treatise is that behavioral patterns of populations and individuals who make up populations are a result of habitual selection from limited choices. She challenged the common notion that a main determinant for unhealthful behavioral choice is lack of knowledge. Governmental and institutional policies, she said set the range of options for personal choice making. It neglected the role of community health nursing, examining the determinants of community health and attempting to influence those determinants through public policy.

Salmon White's Construct for Public Health Nursing

1. Mark Salmon White (1982) describes a public health as an organized societal effort to protect, promote and restore the health of people, and public health nursing as focused on achieving and maintaining public health.
2. He gave three practice priorities, i.e. prevention of disease and poor health, protection against disease, and external agents and promotion of health. For these three general categories of nursing intervention have also been put forward, they are:
   a. Education directed toward voluntary change in the attitude and behavior of the subjects.
   b. Engineering directed at managing risk-related variables.
   c. Enforcement directed at mandatory regulation to achieve better health.

Scope of prevention spans individual, family, community and global care. Intervention target is in four categories:

1. Human/Biological.
2. Environmental.
3. Medical/Technological/Organizational.
4. Social.

Block and Josten's Ethical Theory of Population Focused Nursing

Derryl Block and Lavohn Josten, public health educators proposed this based on intersecting fields of public health and nursing. They have given three essential elements of population focused nursing that stem from these two fields:

1. An obligation to population.
2. The primacy of prevention.
3. Centrality of relationship-based care:
   a. The first two are from public health and the third element from nursing.
   b. Hence it implies to nursing that relation-based care is very important in population focused care.

Canadian Model for Community

The community health nurse works with individuals, families, groups, communities, populations, systems and/or society, but at all times, the health of the person or community is the focus and motivation from which nursing actions flow. The standards of practice are applied to practice in all settings where people live, work, learn, worship and play.

The philosophical base and foundational values, and beliefs that characterize community health nursing care, the principles of primary health care, multiple ways of knowing, individual/community partnerships and empowerment are embedded in the standards and are reflected in the development and application of the community health nursing process.

The community health nursing process involves the traditional nursing process components of assessment, planning, intervention and evaluation, but is enhanced by community health nurses in three dimensions:

1. Individual/Community participation in each component.
2. Multiple ways of knowing, each of which is necessary to understand the complexity and diversity of nursing in the community; knowledge and utilization of all these ways of knowing forms evidence-based practice consistent with these standards.
3. The inherent influence of the broader environment on the individual/community that is the focus of care (e.g. the community will be affected by provincial/territorial policies, its own economic status and by the actions of its individual citizens). The standards of practice are founded on the values and beliefs of community health nurses, and utilization of the community health nursing process.

The model illustrates the dynamic nature of community health nursing practice, embracing the present and projecting into the future. The values and beliefs (green or shaded) ground practice in the present, yet guide the evolution of community health nursing practice overtime. The community health nursing process provides the vehicle through which community health nurses work with people and supports practice that exemplifies the standards of community health nursing. The standards of practice revolve around both the values and beliefs, and the nursing process with the energies of community health nursing always being focused on improving the health of people in the community and facilitating change in systems or society in support of health. Community health nursing practice does not occur in isolation, but rather within an environmental context, such as policies within their workplace and the legislative framework applicable to their work.

FORMULAE FOR CALCULATION OF IMPORTANT VITAL RATES

$$\text{Neonatal mortality} = \frac{\text{No. of infant death of less than 7 days during the year}}{\text{No. of live birth during the year}} \times 100$$

$$\text{Neonatal mortality rate (NMR)} = \frac{\text{No. of infant death of less than 28 days during the year}}{\text{No. of live birth during the year}} \times 100$$

$$\text{Postnatal mortality rate} = \frac{\text{No. of infant death of over 28 days during the year}}{\text{No. of live birth during the year}} \times 100$$

$$\text{Mortality rate (age)} = \frac{\text{No. of death in particular age group}}{\text{Mid-year population of the same age group}} \times 1{,}000$$

$$\text{Maternal mortality rate (MMR)} = \frac{\text{No. of maternal death during the year}}{\text{No. of live birth during the year}} \times 1{,}000$$

$$\text{Infant mortality rate (IME)} = \frac{\text{No. of infant death during the year}}{\text{No. of live birth during the year}} \times 1{,}000$$

$$\text{Stillbirth rate (SBR)} = \frac{\text{No. of stillbirth during the year}}{\text{No. of live birth and stillbirth during the year}} \times 100$$

$$\text{Perinatal mortality rate (PMR)} = \frac{\text{No. of stillbirth and infant deaths}}{\text{No. of live birth and stillbirth during the year}} \times 100$$

$$\text{Crude birth rate (CBR)} = \frac{\text{No. of live birth during the year}}{\text{Mid-year population}} \times 100$$

$$\text{Crude death rate (CDR)} = \frac{\text{No. of death during the year}}{\text{Mid-year population}} \times 100$$

$$\text{Couple protection rate (CPR)} = \frac{\text{No. of eligible couples (ECs) protected either by permanent method or temporary method (RU)}}{\text{Total No. of ECs}} \times 100$$

CLASSIFICATION OF PROTEIN-ENERGY MALNUTRITION

Gomez Classification

Protein-energy malnutrition is graded based on the weight, age as percentage of the expected weight as below:

First degree	Weight between 90 and 75% of expected
Second degree	Weight between 75 and 60% of expected
Third degree	Weight below 60% of expected

Wellcome or International Classification

Weight between 60 and 80% of expected:

With edema	Kwashiorkor
Without edema	Undernutrition

Weight below 60% of expected:

With edema	Marasmic kwashiorkor
Without edema	Nutritional marasmus

Classification of Indian Academy of Pediatrics

First degree	Weight between 80 and 70% of expected
Second degree	Weight between 70 and 60% of expected
Third degree	Weight between 60 and 50% of expected
Fourth degree	Weight below 50% of expected

In case if the patient has demonstrable edema, the letter 'K' is placed in front of the evaluated grade.

Jelliffe Classification

First degree	Weight between 90 and 80% of expected
Second degree	Weight between 80 and 70% of expected
Third degree	Weight between 70 and 60% of expected
Fourth degree	Weight below 60% of expected

McLaren Classification

Mild	Weight between 90 and 80% of expected
Moderate	Weight between 80 and 70% of expected
Severe	Weight below 70% of expected

Arnold Classification

It is based on mid-arm circumference (MAC) as follows:

Mild to moderate	MAC between 12.5 and 13.5 cm
Severe	MAC under 12.5 cm

Classification Based on Skin Fold Thickness

Mild	80–90% of expected
Moderate	60–80%
Severe	Under 60%

Recommended dietary allowance (RDA) for Indians

Group	Particulars	Body weight (kg)	Net Energy (kcal/d)	Protein (g/d)	Fat (g/d)	Calcium (mg/d)	Iron (mg/d)	Vitamin A (mg/d)		Thiamine (mg/d)	Riboflavin (mg/d)	Nicotinic acid (mg/d)	Pyridoxine (mg/d)	Ascorbic acid (mg/d)	Folic acid (mg/d)	Vitamin B_{12} (mg/d)
								Retinol	β-carotene							
Woman	Pregnant Women Lactation	50	+300	+15	30	1,000	38	600	2,400	+0.2	+0.2	+2	2.5	40	400	1
Infant	0.6 month	50	+500	+25						+0.3	4 +		2.5	80		
	6–12 month		+400	+18	45	1,000	30	950	3,800	+0.2	+0.2	+3			150	1.5
	0–6 month	5.4	108/kg	2.5/kg						55 mg/kg	65 mg/kg	170 mg/kg	0.1			
	6–12 month	8.6	98/kg	1.65/kg		500		350	1,200	50 mg/kg	60 mg/kg	650 mg/kg	0.4	25	25	0.2
Children	1–3 year	12.2	1,240	22			12	400		0.6	0.7	8			30	
	4–6 year	19.0	1,690	30	25	400	18	400	1,600	0.9	1.0	11	0.9	40	40	0.2–10
	7–9 year	26.9	1,950	41			26	600	12,400	1.0	1.2	13	1.6		60	

Group	Particulars	Body weight (kg)	Net energy (kcal/d)	Protein (g/d)	Fat (g/d)	Calcium (mg/d)	Iron (mg/d)	Vitamin A (mg/d)		Thiamine (mg/d)	Riboflavin (mg/d)	Nicotinic acid (mg/d)	Pyridoxine (mg/d)	Ascorbic acid (mg/d)	Folic acid (mg/d)	Vitamin B_{12} (mg/d)
								Retinol	β-carotene							
Boys	10–12 year	35.4	2,190	54			64			1.1	1.3	15				
Girls	10–12 year	31.5	1,970	57	22	600	19	600	2,400	1.0	1.2	13	1.6	40	70	0.2–1.0
Boys	13–15 year	47.8	2,450	70			41			1.2	1.5	16				
Girls	13–15 year	46.7	2,060	65	22	600	28	600	2,400	1.0	1.2	14	2.0	20	100	0.2–1.0
Boys	16–18 year	57.1	2,640	78			50			1.3	1.6	17				
Girls	16–18 year	49.9	2,060	63	22	600	30	600	2,400	1.0	1.2	14	2.0	20	100	0.2–1.0

WHO recommended nutritive values for commonly used food items in India

Sl No.	Food preparation	Quantity per serving	Weight per serving	Calories (kcal)	Protein (g)	Fat (g)	Carbohydrates (g)	Calcium (g)	Phosphorus (g)	Iron (mg)
Cereal and millet preparation										
I	*Rice preparation*									
1.	Plain rice	2 serving	504	595	11.9	0.9	134.8	0.02	0.2	11.9
2.	Sambar rice	1 serving	485	405	13.5	13.5	76.2	0.08	0.16	13.5
3.	Curd rice	1 serving	253	221	6	7	33.3	0.57	0.10	6
4.	Sweet rice	1 serving	177	432	3.6	12	77.4	0.01	0.05	3.6
5.	Idli	2 pcs	136	130	4.6	0.2	27.6	0.03	0.08	4.6
6.	Plain dosa	2 pcs	100	216	4.1	9.7	28.2	0.03	0.07	4 1
7.	Masala dosa	2 pcs	100	212	4.6	8 4	29.4	0.04	0.08	4.6
8.	Pongal (hot)	1 serving	148	200	5.5	6	30.5	0.03	0.07	5.5
9.	Adai (hot)	1 pc	96	195	6.6	4.4	31.8	0.03	0.09	6.6
II	*Wheat preparation*									
1.	Wheat upma	1 serving	128	163	3.8	5.4	24.7	0.01	0.04	0.7
2.	Chapatis	2 pcs	57	196	5	5.5	30.8	0.13	0.02	3
3.	Puris	2 pcs	32	136	2.2	8.4	13	0.06	0.01	1.3
4.	Plain parathas	1 pc	66	104	4.5	19.6	27.3	0.12	0.01	2.7
5.	Rava (dosa, idli)	2 pcs	114	212	5	8.5	28.7	0	0.06	0.9
6.	Kesari bath	1 serving	90	284	2	14.6	35.3	0.02	0.04	0.44
7.	Luchi	2 pcs	71	346	4	24	28	0.03	0.01	0.4
III	*Millet preparation*									
1.	Ragi balls	1 pc	336	446	6	7.6	86.8	0.3	0.4	6
2.	Ragi roti	2 pcs	185	460	8	9	87	0.3	0.4	6
3.	Maize roti	2 pcs	142	314	9.6	5.5	56.4	0.3	0.1	1.8
4.	Jowar roti	2 pcs	150	252	7.5	1.3	52.5	0.2	0.02	4.5
5.	Ragi puttu	1 serving	146	422	4.4	7.4	84	0.2	0.02	
IV	*Pulse preparation*									
1.	Bengal gram dal (cooked)	1½ cup	157	284	9	16.4	25.2	0.07	0.13	3.8
2.	Bengal gram dal	1 cup	154	178	3.2	35.9	44.7	0.09	0.08	0.4
3.	Green gram dal (cooked)	1½ cup	142	171	7	7.7	18.4	0.08	0.09	2.7
4.	Red gram dal (cooked)	1½ cup	96	110	6.4	2	16.4	0.05	0.07	2.6
5.	Dal rasam	1½ cup	196	29	1.5	0.9	3.8	0.03	0.03	0.09
6.	Radish sambar (sundal)		196	101	4.1	3.6	13.1	0.04	0.07	2.2
7.	Green gram sambar (sundal)	1 cup	142	255	13.5	8.8	30.3	0.05	0.2	2.5

Contd...

Contd...

Sl No.	Food preparation	Quantity per serving	Weight per serving	Calories (kcal)	Protein (g)	Fat (g)	Carbohydrates (g)	Calcium (g)	Phosphorus (g)	Iron (mg)
8.	Cowpea sundal	1 cup	142	259	13.1	9.2	30.9	0.08	0.2	4.8
9.	Amaranth sambar	1½ cup	140	250	5.1	2.7	13	0.05	0.08	8
10.	Bengal gram (sundal)	1 cup	142	272	13.2	11.1	29.7	0.11	0.15	5.5
V	*Vegetable preparation*									
1.	Amaranth curry	1½ plate	28	47	1.4	2.3	5.1	0.04	0.04	6.64
2.	Amaranth masala	½ plate	42	46	1.2	2.6	4.4	0.05	0.05	6.8
3.	Brinjal curry	½ plate	45	122	1.4	10.7	4.9	0.02	0.05	0.9
4.	Milk (buffalo)	1 cup	200	216	8.4	16	9.2	0.42	0.030	0.8
5.	Cabbage and carrot curry	½ plate	56	81	1.5	5.6	6.1	0.04	0.12	0.9
6.	Buttermilk	1 cup	200	36	1.8	2.8	2	0.07	0.07	0.2
7.	Buttermilk (buffalo)	1 cup	200	66	24	5.4	2.8	0.07	0.07	0.2
VI	*Egg, milk and meat preparation*									
1.	Meat curry	1 serving	128	220	116	18	2.7	0.1	0.01	2.1
2.	Omelet	1 serving	39	77	5.8	5.7	0.5	0.03	0.1	1
3.	Meat fry	1 serving	142	339	21.8	26	4.5	0.23	0.2	3.3
4.	Fish fry	1 serving	100	220	16.2	16.2	1.4	0.05	0.45	1.2
5.	Rice, mutton pulao	2 servings	341	686	39	39	63.6	0.1	0.22	1.5
VII	*Preparation containing milk*									
1.	Coffee	1 cup	200	104	3.8	3.4	14.4	0.1	0.1	1.2
2.	Tea	1 cup	200	72	1.4	1.6	13	0.06	0.04	-
3.	Cocoa	1 cup	200	174	7.5	20.2	20.2	0.2	0.15	0.3
4.	Wheat payasam	1 cup	154	178	3.4	31.5	31.5	0.09	0.08	0.4
5.	Rice payasam	1 cup	266	227	3.7	44.3	44.3	0.14	0.1	4.7
6.	Rice porridge	1 cup	280	263	7.6	44.7	35.9	0.3	0.2	0.7
7.	Soy porridge	1 cup	154	178	7.7	44	44.7	0.07	0.14	0.4
8.	Wheat porridge	1 cup	280	263	7.6	44.7	35.9	0.3	0.22	0.7
9.	Ragi porridge	1 cup	193	317	8.7	52.7	35.9	0.24	0.22	1
10.	Milk (cow)	1 cup	200	130	7	9.8	52.7	0.12	0.1	0.4

Practical Experience of Community Health Nursing Program Schedule

Name of the Student : ____________________

Community Area : ____________________

Name of the Clinical Instructor : ____________________

Sl No.	Date	Activities

Sl No.	Date	Activities

Signature of the Clinical Coordinator
Date:

Signature of the HOD of Community Health Nursing
Date:

Signature of the Principal
Date:

Orientation Report

Time Schedule and Introduction of Orientation

Members of Group

Numbers of Group

Requesting Permission from Medical Officer

Distance Between College and PHC, PHC to Village

Identification of PHC and Route Map of PHC

Total Number of Houses

Total Population

Area

Landmarks

Specify the Religious Places

Area Map

Signature of the Clinical Instructor
Date:

Signature of HOD of Community Health Nursing
Date:

Primary Health Center Report

Introduction

Name of the Primary Health Center (PHC)

Functions of PHC

Staffing Pattern in PHC

Special Days in PHC

Drugs and Equipment, Supplies in PHC

Floor Map

Note: During posting, students' observance has to be written as a PHC report.

Community Survey Assessment

Identification Data

1. Name of the Area (Rural/Urban): __________
2. House Number: __________
3. Name of the Health Center: __________
4. Name of Head of the Family: __________
5. Family Identification: __________
   a. Total number of members in the family: __________
   b. Type of family (nuclear/joint/extended): __________
   c. Religion (Hindu/Muslim/Christian/others): __________
   d. Specify subcaste: __________
   e. Language known: __________
   f. Statement of expenditure of the family:

Items	Amount spent	Expenditure in %	Items	Amount spent	Expenditure in %
Food			Clothing		
House rent			Medicine		
Children education			Recreation (movies, etc.)		
Smoking and liquor			Debt		
Savings			Others (specify)		
			Total		

6. Housing Condition: __________
   a. Type of house:
      Kutcha: __________ Pucca: __________ Semi-pucca: __________
   b. Living rooms:
      Number: __________ Adequate: __________ Inadequate: __________
   c. Occupancy: __________
      Tenant: __________ Owner: __________ Monthly rent: __________

d. Ventilation: ______

Adequate: ______ Inadequate: ______ No ventilation: ______

e. Source of lighting: ______

Electricity: ______ Kerosene: ______ Others (specify): ______

f. Water supply: ______

Tube well: ______ Dug well: ______ Lake: ______ Pond: ______

Municipality water: ______ Others: ______

g. Kitchen condition: ______

Separate: ______ Corner of the house: ______ Veranda: ______

h. Disposal of waste: ______

Open dumping: ______ Incineration: ______ Manure pits: ______ Others: ______

i. Sullage water disposal:

Open drainage: ______ Closed drain: ______ Soakage pit: ______ Kitchen garden: ______

ii. Refuse disposal:

Indiscriminate throwing: ______ Garbage: ______ Compositing: ______

Burning: ______ Municipal collection: ______ Dumping: ______

iii. Excreta disposal:

Open air defecation: ______ Separate latrine: ______ Shared latrine: ______

Public toilet: ______

7. Family Profile:

Sl No.	Name of the family member	Relation with head of the family	Age in year	Sex	Education	Occupation	Income	Remark on health
1.								
2.								
3.								
4.								
5.								
6.								
7.								

a. Total family income per month/year: ₹ ______

8. Transport and Communication:

a. Transport:

i. Own tempo/tractor: ______

ii. Use government bus: ______

iii. Any other: ______

b. Communication:

   i. Telephone: ____________

   ii. Television: ____________

   iii. Radio: ____________

   iv. Newspaper/Magazine: ____________

   v. Post and telegraph: ____________

9. Dietary Pattern:

Food	Food used	Food preparation and storage		
		Traditional	Ideal	Unhygienic
Rice				
Ragi				
Jawar				
Wheat				
Vegetable				
Fish				
Meat				
Egg				
Milk and products				
Pulses				
Tubers				
Any others specify				

10. Nutritional Status:

Name	Weight (kg)	Height (cm)	Body built				BMI (normal 19–25)		
			Thin	Moderate	Well	Obese	Normal	< normal	> normal

a. Nutritional deficiency:

Anemic: ____________ Goiter: ____________ Night blindness: ____________

Scurvy: ____________ Rickets: ____________ Others: ____________

11. Is there any case of fever (if yes, write name, age, treatment with remarks):
    a. With rigors.
    b. With cough.
    c. With rash.

Sl No.	Name	Age	Discuss	Treatment	Remarks
1.					
2.					
3.					

12. Does anyone have any skin disease (e.g. itching, patch, rash)?

Sl No.	Name	Age	Discuss	Treatment	Remarks
1.					
2.					
3.					

13. Does anyone have cough more than 1 week?

Sl No.	Name	Age	Discuss	Treatment	Remarks
1.					
2.					
3.					

14. Does anyone have any other illness?

Sl No.	Name	Age	Discuss	Treatment	Remarks
1.					
2.					
3.					

15. Is there any woman pregnant? If yes, write the following remarks:
    a. Specify gravida.
    b. Has she been registered?
    c. Is she getting iron and folic acid?
    d. Has she had tetanus toxoid?

Sl No.	Name	Age	Discuss	Treatment	Remarks
1.					
2.					
3.					

16. Have there been any (within year) vital statistics?
    a. Births?

Sl No.	Date of birth	Sex	Parents name	Remarks
1.				
2.				
3.				

    b. Deaths?

Sl No.	Date of death	Sex	Parents name	Remarks
1.				
2.				
3.				

    c. Marriages?

Sl No.	Date of marriage	Sex	Spouse name	Remarks
1.				
2.				
3.				

17. Are there any children below 5 years who have not received immunization? (Specify name, age, reasons for not immunized in remarks):
    a. Bacillus Calmette-Guérin (BCG) vaccination.
    b. Diphtheria, pertussis and tetanus (DPT) vaccination.
    c. Poliomyelitis vaccination.
    d. Measles vaccination.
    e. Vitamin A solution.

Sl No.	Name	Age	Sex	17a	17b			17c	17c	17e
					1	2	3			

18. Presence of the following:
    a. Mosquitoes: ______________ House fly: ______________
    b. Stray dogs: ______________ Cats: ______________ Specify number: ______________

c. Accident place (environment):

Sharp stones: ________ Slippery floor: ________ Stones: ________

Open drainage: ________ Others (specify): ________

Signature of the Clinical Instructor
Date:

Signature of HOD of Community Health Nursing
Date:

Household Survey

Case 1

House Number : ____________________

Name of the Village : ____________________

Name of the Street : ____________________

Name of Head of the Family : ____________________

Name of the Informer : ____________________

Religion : ____________________

Caste : ____________________

Type of Family : ____________________

Economic Status : ____________________

Environmental Sanitation : ____________________

Water Supply : Adequate/Inadequate

Water Supply : Tank/Well/Hand pump

Water Supply : Protected/Unprotected

Refuse Disposal : Open dumping/Burning/Manure pit

Waste Water Disposal : ____________________ Stagnation: Yes/No: ____________

If yes, Mention Type : ____________________

Excreta Disposal : ____________________ Latrine: Yes/No: ____________

If yes, Mention Type : ____________________

Particular of the household member

Sl No.	Name of the family member	Relation to the head of the family	Age/Sex	Marital status	Education status	Occupation status	Income	Residential status	Health status	Remarks

VITAL STATISTICS

Birth status

Sl No.	Name of the child/Name of the parent	Date of birth/Sex	Place of birth	Whether registered	Delivery conducted	Health status of the child	Remarks

Death status

Sl No.	Name of the deceased person	Age/Sex	Date of death	Place of death	Whether registered	Cause of death	Remarks

Family welfare—maternal and child health

Sl No.	Name of the eligible	Age at marriage/ whether registered	Pregnancy status/ number of pregnancy	Type of delivery	Baby alive/ dead	Age of the child/sex of the baby	Birth weight of the baby	Term/ Abortion	Any congenital deformities	Remarks

Signature of the Student
Date:

Signature of the Clinical Instructor
Date:

Household Survey

Case 2

House Number	: ______________________
Name of the Village	: ______________________
Name of the Street	: ______________________
Name of Head of the Family	: ______________________
Name of the Informer	: ______________________
Religion	: ______________________
Caste	: ______________________
Type of Family	: ______________________
Economic Status	: ______________________
Environmental Sanitation	: ______________________
Water Supply	: Adequate/Inadequate
Water Supply	: Tank/Well/Hand pump
Water Supply	: Protected/Unprotected
Refuse Disposal	: Open dumping/Burning/Manure pit
Waste Water Disposal	: ______________ Stagnation: Yes/No: ________
If yes, Mention Type	: ______________________
Excreta Disposal	: ______________ Latrine: Yes/No: ________
If yes, Mention Type	: ______________________

Particular of the household member

Sl No.	Name of the family member	Relation to the head of the family	Age/Sex	Marital status	Education status	Occupation status	Income	Residential status	Health status	Remarks

VITAL STATISTICS

Birth status

Sl No.	Name of the child/Name of the parent	Date of birth/Sex	Place of birth	Whether registered	Delivery conducted	Health status of the child	Remarks

Death status

Sl No.	Name of the deceased person	Age/Sex	Date of death	Place of death	Whether registered	Cause of death	Remarks

Family welfare—maternal and child health

Sl No.	Name of the eligible	Age at marriage/ whether registered	Pregnancy status/ number of pregnancy	Type of delivery	Baby alive/ dead	Age of the child/sex of the baby	Birth weight of the baby	Term/ Abortion	Any congenital deformities	Remarks

Signature of the Student
Date:

Signature of the Clinical Instructor
Date:

Household Survey

Case 3

House Number : ____________________

Name of the Village : ____________________

Name of the Street : ____________________

Name of Head of the Family : ____________________

Name of the Informer : ____________________

Religion : ____________________

Caste : ____________________

Type of Family : ____________________

Economic Status : ____________________

Environmental Sanitation : ____________________

Water Supply : Adequate/Inadequate

Water Supply : Tank/Well/Hand pump

Water Supply : Protected/Unprotected

Refuse Disposal : Open dumping/Burning/Manure pit

Waste Water Disposal : ____________________ Stagnation: Yes/No: ____________

If yes, Mention Type : ____________________

Excreta Disposal : ____________________ Latrine: Yes/No: ____________

If yes, Mention Type : ____________________

Particular of the household member

Sl No.	Name of the family member	Relation to the head of the family	Age/Sex	Marital status	Education status	Occupation status	Income	Residential status	Health status	Remarks

VITAL STATISTICS

Birth status

Sl No.	Name of the child/Name of the parent	Date of birth/Sex	Place of birth	Whether registered	Delivery conducted	Health status of the child	Remarks

Death status

Sl No.	Name of the deceased person	Age/Sex	Date of death	Place of death	Whether registered	Cause of death	Remarks

Family welfare—maternal and child health

Sl No.	Name of the eligible	Age at marriage/ whether registered	Pregnancy status/ number of pregnancy	Type of delivery	Baby alive/ dead	Age of the child/sex of the baby	Birth weight of the baby	Term/ Abortion	Any congenital deformities	Remarks

Signature of the Student
Date:

Signature of the Clinical Instructor
Date:

Household Survey

Case 4

House Number : ____________________

Name of the Village : ____________________

Name of the Street : ____________________

Name of Head of the Family : ____________________

Name of the Informer : ____________________

Religion : ____________________

Caste : ____________________

Type of Family : ____________________

Economic Status : ____________________

Environmental Sanitation : ____________________

Water Supply : Adequate/Inadequate

Water Supply : Tank/Well/Hand pump

Water Supply : Protected/Unprotected

Refuse Disposal : Open dumping/Burning/Manure pit

Waste Water Disposal : ____________________ Stagnation: Yes/No: __________

If yes, Mention Type : ____________________

Excreta Disposal : ____________________ Latrine: Yes/No: __________

If yes, Mention Type : ____________________

Particular of the household member

Sl No.	Name of the family member	Relation to the head of the family	Age/Sex	Marital status	Education status	Occupation status	Income	Residential status	Health status	Remarks

VITAL STATISTICS

Birth status

Sl No.	Name of the child/Name of the parent	Date of birth/Sex	Place of birth	Whether registered	Delivery conducted	Health status of the child	Remarks

Death status

Sl No.	Name of the deceased person	Age/Sex	Date of death	Place of death	Whether registered	Cause of death	Remarks

Family welfare—maternal and child health

Sl No.	Name of the eligible	Age at marriage/ whether registered	Pregnancy status/ number of pregnancy	Type of delivery	Baby alive/ dead	Age of the child/sex of the baby	Birth weight of the baby	Term/ Abortion	Any congenital deformities	Remarks

Signature of the Student
Date:

Signature of the Clinical Instructor
Date:

Household Survey

Case 5

House Number : ____________________
Name of the Village : ____________________
Name of the Street : ____________________
Name of Head of the Family : ____________________
Name of the Informer : ____________________
Religion : ____________________
Caste : ____________________
Type of Family : ____________________
Economic Status : ____________________
Environmental Sanitation : ____________________
Water Supply : Adequate/Inadequate
Water Supply : Tank/Well/Hand pump
Water Supply : Protected/Unprotected
Refuse Disposal : Open dumping/Burning/Manure pit
Waste Water Disposal : ____________________ Stagnation: Yes/No: ____________
If yes, Mention Type : ____________________
Excreta Disposal : ____________________ Latrine: Yes/No: ____________
If yes, Mention Type : ____________________

Particular of the household member

Sl No.	Name of the family member	Relation to the head of the family	Age/Sex	Marital status	Education status	Occupation status	Income	Residential status	Health status	Remarks

VITAL STATISTICS

Birth status

Sl No.	Name of the child/Name of the parent	Date of birth/Sex	Place of birth	Whether registered	Delivery conducted	Health status of the child	Remarks

Death status

Sl No.	Name of the deceased person	Age/Sex	Date of death	Place of death	Whether registered	Cause of death	Remarks

Family welfare—maternal and child health

Sl No.	Name of the eligible	Age at marriage/ whether registered	Pregnancy status/ number of pregnancy	Type of delivery	Baby alive/ dead	Age of the child/sex of the baby	Birth weight of the baby	Term/ Abortion	Any congenital deformities	Remarks

Signature of the Student
Date:

Signature of the Clinical Instructor
Date:

Family Folder

Case 1

Identification Data

Name of the Area (Rural/Urban): __________

House Number: __________

Name of the Health Center: __________

Name of Head of the Family: __________

Family Identification: __________

Total Number of Members in the Family: __________

Type of Family (Nuclear/Nonnuclear): __________

Religion (Hindu/Muslim/Christian/Others): __________

Specify Subcaste: __________

Language Known: __________

Name of the Informer: __________

Age/Sex: __________

Address: __________

Education Status: __________

Occupational Status: __________

Income of the Family: ₹ __________/month

Family Composition

Sl No.	Name of the family members	Age	Sex	Relationship with head of the family	Education status	Occupation status	Health status
1.							
2.							
3.							
4.							

Contd...

Contd...

Sl No.	Name of the family members	Age	Sex	Relationship with head of the family	Education status	Occupation status	Health status
5.							
6.							
7.							
8.							
9.							
10.							
11.							
12.							

Immunization Chart

Sl No.	Immunization schedule	Due date	Given date	Weight of the baby/Advice
1.	At birth BCG, OPV-0			
2.	45 day DPT, OPV-1			
3.	75 day DPT, OPV-2			
4.	105 day DPT, OPV-3			
5.	9–10 month measles			
6.	18 month DPT, OPV booster dose			
7.	5 year DT, OPV			
8.	10 year TT			
9.	Optional vaccines			
10.				
11.				

Past History of Illness

____

____

____

____

____

Present Complaints

List Out the Problems and Needs

1.
2.
3.
4.
5.
6.

Problems/Needs	Objectives	Nursing interventions	Rationale	Evaluations

Contd...

Contd...

Problems/Needs	Objectives	Nursing interventions	Rationale	Evaluations

Contd...

Contd...

Problems/Needs	Objectives	Nursing interventions	Rationale	Evaluations

Contd...

Contd...

Problems/Needs	Objectives	Nursing interventions	Rationale	Evaluations

Family Folder

Case 2

Identification Data

Name of the Area (Rural/Urban): ______

House Number: ______

Name of the Health Center: ______

Name of Head of the Family: ______

Family Identification: ______

Total Number of Members in the Family: ______

Type of Family (Nuclear/Nonnuclear): ______

Religion (Hindu/Muslim/Christian/Others): ______

Specify Subcaste: ______

Language Known: ______

Name of the Informer: ______

Age/Sex: ______

Address: ______

______

______

______

Education Status: ______

Occupational Status: ______

Income of the Family: ₹ ______/month

Family Composition

Sl No.	Name of the family members	Age	Sex	Relationship with head of the family	Education status	Occupation status	Health status
1.							
2.							
3.							
4.							

Contd...

Contd...

Sl No.	Name of the family members	Age	Sex	Relationship with head of the family	Education status	Occupation status	Health status
5.							
6.							
7.							
8.							
9.							
10.							
11.							
12.							

Immunization Chart

Sl No.	Immunization schedule	Due date	Given date	Weight of the baby/Advice
1.	At birth BCG, OPV-0			
2.	45 day DPT, OPV-1			
3.	75 day DPT, OPV-2			
4.	105 day DPT, OPV-3			
5.	9–10 month measles			
6.	18 month DPT, OPV booster dose			
7.	5 year DT, OPV			
8.	10 year TT			
9.	Optional vaccines			
10.				
11.				

Past History of Illness

____

____

____

____

____

Present Complaints

List Out the Problems and Needs

1.
2.
3.
4.
5.
6.

Problems/Needs	Objectives	Nursing interventions	Rationale	Evaluations

Contd...

Contd...

Problems/Needs	Objectives	Nursing interventions	Rationale	Evaluations

Contd...

Contd...

Problems/Needs	Objectives	Nursing interventions	Rationale	Evaluations

Contd...

Contd...

Problems/Needs	Objectives	Nursing interventions	Rationale	Evaluations

Family Folder

Case 3

Identification Data

Name of the Area (Rural/Urban): ____________________

House Number: ____________________

Name of the Health Center: ____________________

Name of Head of the Family: ____________________

Family Identification: ____________________

Total Number of Members in the Family: ____________________

Type of Family (Nuclear/Nonnuclear): ____________________

Religion (Hindu/Muslim/Christian/Others): ____________________

Specify Subcaste: ____________________

Language Known: ____________________

Name of the Informer: ____________________

Age/Sex: ____________________

Address: ____________________

____

____

____

Education Status: ____________________

Occupational Status: ____________________

Income of the Family: ₹ ____________________/month

Family Composition

Sl No.	Name of the family members	Age	Sex	Relationship with head of the family	Education status	Occupation status	Health status
1.							
2.							
3.							
4.							

Contd...

Contd...

Sl No.	Name of the family members	Age	Sex	Relationship with head of the family	Education status	Occupation status	Health status
5.							
6.							
7.							
8.							
9.							
10.							
11.							
12.							

Immunization Chart

Sl No.	Immunization schedule	Due date	Given date	Weight of the baby/Advice
1.	At birth BCG, OPV-0			
2.	45 day DPT, OPV-1			
3.	75 day DPT, OPV-2			
4.	105 day DPT, OPV-3			
5.	9–10 month measles			
6.	18 month DPT, OPV booster dose			
7.	5 year DT, OPV			
8.	10 year TT			
9.	Optional vaccines			
10.				
11.				

Past History of Illness

____

____

____

____

____

Present Complaints

List Out the Problems and Needs

1.
2.
3.
4.
5.
6.

Problems/Needs	Objectives	Nursing interventions	Rationale	Evaluations

Contd...

Contd...

Problems/Needs	Objectives	Nursing interventions	Rationale	Evaluations

Contd...

Contd...

Problems/Needs	Objectives	Nursing interventions	Rationale	Evaluations

Contd...

Contd...

Problems/Needs	Objectives	Nursing interventions	Rationale	Evaluations

Family Folder

Case 4

Identification Data

Name of the Area (Rural/Urban): ____________________

House Number: ____________________

Name of the Health Center: ____________________

Name of Head of the Family: ____________________

Family Identification: ____________________

Total Number of Members in the Family: ____________________

Type of Family (Nuclear/Nonnuclear): ____________________

Religion (Hindu/Muslim/Christian/Others): ____________________

Specify Subcaste: ____________________

Language Known: ____________________

Name of the Informer: ____________________

Age/Sex: ____________________

Address: ____________________

____

____

____

Education Status: ____________________

Occupational Status: ____________________

Income of the Family: ₹ ____________________/month

Family Composition

Sl No.	Name of the family members	Age	Sex	Relationship with head of the family	Education status	Occupation status	Health status
1.							
2.							
3.							
4.							

Contd...

Contd...

Sl No.	Name of the family members	Age	Sex	Relationship with head of the family	Education status	Occupation status	Health status
5.							
6.							
7.							
8.							
9.							
10.							
11.							
12.							

Immunization Chart

Sl No.	Immunization schedule	Due date	Given date	Weight of the baby/Advice
1.	At birth BCG, OPV-0			
2.	45 day DPT, OPV-1			
3.	75 day DPT, OPV-2			
4.	105 day DPT, OPV-3			
5.	9–10 month measles			
6.	18 month DPT, OPV booster dose			
7.	5 year DT, OPV			
8.	10 year TT			
9.	Optional vaccines			
10.				
11.				

Past History of Illness

____

____

____

____

____

Present Complaints

List Out the Problems and Needs

1.
2.
3.
4.
5.
6.

Problems/Needs	Objectives	Nursing interventions	Rationale	Evaluations

Contd...

Contd...

Problems/Needs	Objectives	Nursing interventions	Rationale	Evaluations

Contd...

Contd...

Problems/Needs	Objectives	Nursing interventions	Rationale	Evaluations

Contd...

Contd...

Problems/Needs	Objectives	Nursing interventions	Rationale	Evaluations

Family Folder

Case 5

Identification Data

Name of the Area (Rural/Urban): __________

House Number: __________

Name of the Health Center: __________

Name of Head of the Family: __________

Family Identification: __________

Total Number of Members in the Family: __________

Type of Family (Nuclear/Nonnuclear): __________

Religion (Hindu/Muslim/Christian/Others): __________

Specify Subcaste: __________

Language Known: __________

Name of the Informer: __________

Age/Sex: __________

Address: __________

Education Status: __________

Occupational Status: __________

Income of the Family: ₹ __________/month

Family Composition

Sl No.	Name of the family members	Age	Sex	Relationship with head of the family	Education status	Occupation status	Health status
1.							
2.							
3.							
4.							

Contd...

Contd...

Sl No.	Name of the family members	Age	Sex	Relationship with head of the family	Education status	Occupation status	Health status
5.							
6.							
7.							
8.							
9.							
10.							
11.							
12.							

Immunization Chart

Sl No.	Immunization schedule	Due date	Given date	Weight of the baby/Advice
1.	At birth BCG, OPV-0			
2.	45 day DPT, OPV-1			
3.	75 day DPT, OPV-2			
4.	105 day DPT, OPV-3			
5.	9–10 month measles			
6.	18 month DPT, OPV booster dose			
7.	5 year DT, OPV			
8.	10 year TT			
9.	Optional vaccines			
10.				
11.				

Past History of Illness

____

____

____

____

____

Present Complaints

List Out the Problems and Needs

1.
2.
3.
4.
5.
6.

Problems/Needs	Objectives	Nursing interventions	Rationale	Evaluations

Contd...

Contd...

Problems/Needs	Objectives	Nursing interventions	Rationale	Evaluations

Contd...

Contd...

Problems/Needs	Objectives	Nursing interventions	Rationale	Evaluations

Contd...

Contd...

Problems/Needs	Objectives	Nursing interventions	Rationale	Evaluations

Family Care Plan

Case 1

Identification Data

House Number: ____________________

Name of the Informer: ____________________

Age: ____________________

Sex: ____________________

Name of Head of the Family: ____________________

Address: ____________________

____

____

____

Type of Family: ____________________

Family Size: ____________________

Religion: ____________________

Caste: ____________________

Educational Status: ____________________

Occupational Status: ____________________

Income of the Family: ₹ ____________________/month

Mother Tongue: ____________________

Student Data

Name of the Student: ____________________

Course: ____________________

Class: ____________________

Date of Care Started: ____________________

Date of Care Ended: ____________________

Family Composition

Sl No.	Name of the family members	Age	Sex	Relationship with head of the family	Education status	Occupation status	Health status
1.							
2.							
3.							
4.							
5.							
6.							
7.							

Socioeconomic Status

Family Tree

Past Medical History

Past Surgical History

Present History of Illness

Housing Pattern (Floor Map)

Housing and Environmental Condition

Type of house	:	
Roof	:	Thatch/Thatti/Tilled/Terraced/Others
Floor	:	Mud/Tiled/Cemented/Others
Wall	:	Thatti/Mud/Brick/Cement plastered/Others
Housing pattern	:	Pucca/Semi-pucca/Kutcha/Others
Possession	:	Own house/Rental house/Leased
Area (square feet)	:	Adequate/Inadequate
Ventilation	:	Natural/Artificial
Number of rooms	:	
Doors/Windows	:	Adequate/Inadequate
Electricity	:	Available/Not available
Mode of lighting	:	Oil lamp/Kerosene/Electric bulb/Others
Water supply	:	Adequate/Inadequate
Mode of water supply	:	Well/Public tap/Hand pump/Others
Latrine	:	Service/Water seal/Open field
Drain	:	Open/Closed/Nil
Street light	:	Yes/No
Street road condition	:	Cement/Tar/Mud/Others
Type of fuel used	:	Firewood/Kerosene/Gas/Cow dung/Biogas
Open space around the house	:	Yes/No
Garden	:	Yes/No
Water stagnation	:	Yes/No
Disposal of waste	:	Drum/Open space/Manure pit/Burning/Throwing into street/Separate
Livestock and poultry	:	Available/Not available
If available	:	Shed/Separate
	:	Attached/Mixed
Healthcare facilities	:	GH/PHC/SC/Private doctors/Others
Medical aid available in the street	:	Doctor/Homeo/Siddha/Village vaidyas/Others
Playground in the street	:	Available/Not available
Social institution	:	Bank/Post office/Police station/Market/Transport
Educational institution	:	Primary school/Secondary school/HSS/College/Night school/Adult school/Crèche
Religious institution	:	Temple/Church/Mosque/Others
Presence of rodents	:	
Presence of stray dog	:	
Presence of domestic animals	:	
Presence of insects	:	

Economical Status

Income : ____________________/month
Source of income : ____________________
Number of earning members : ____________________
Expenditure : ____________________/month
Rent : ____________________/month
Food : ____________________/month
Health : ____________________/month
School : ____________________/month
Miscellaneous : ____________________/month
Own properties : Land/Vehicle/House/Others

Transportation

Bus : ____________________; specify, which bus: ____________________
Auto rickshaw : ____________________ Yes/No
Four wheelers : ____________________ Yes/No
Train : ____________________ Yes/No
Airway : ____________________ Yes/No

Communication

Face to face : ____________________
Mobile : ____________________
Telephone : ____________________
Through letter : ____________________
Internet : ____________________

Personal hobbies

Recreational activity : ____________________

Nutritional Status of Family

Dietary pattern : Vegetarian/Nonvegetarian/Ovo vegetarian
Frequency of nonvegetarian : ____________________
Food habit: Number of meals : ____________________/day
Cooking method : ____________________
Staple food : ____________________
Sources of food items
(vegetables) : ____________________
Storage of food items : ____________________
Usage of processed food items : ____________________

Beneficiary data

Name of beneficiary : ____________________

Age : ____________________

Sex : ____________________

Menu plan

Sl No.	Type of food	Amount of food	Calories (kcal)
Breakfast			
1.			
2.			
Midmorning			
1.			
2.			
Lunch			
1.			
2.			
3.			
Evening			
1.			
2.			
Dinner			
1.			
2.			
3.			
		Total	

Amount allotted for nutrition : ____________________

Use of:

- Vegetables : ____________________
- Fruits : ____________________
- Cereals/Pulses/Nuts : ____________________

Plan for Home Visit

Sl No.	Name of the beneficiary	Date	Needs/Problems	Preventions	Short-term goals	Long-term goals

Physical Examination

General appearance

Nourishment : ______________________

Body built : ______________________

Health : ______________________

Activity : ______________________

Mental status

Consciousness : ______________________

Look : ______________________

Vital signs

Temperature : ______________________°C

Pulse : ______________________/minute

Respiration : ______________________/minute

Blood pressure : ______________________mm Hg

Anthropometric measurement

Height or length (cm) : ______________________

Weight (kg) : ______________________

Chest circumference (cm) : ______________________

Mid-arm circumference (cm) : ______________________

Body mass index (BMI) : ______________________

Skin condition : ______________________

Color : ______________________

Texture : ______________________

Lesion : ______________________

Sensation : ______________________

Head and face

Scalp : ______________________

Face : ______________________

Hair color : ______________________

Eye

Eyebrows : ______________________

Eyelashes : ______________________

Eyelids : ______________________

Eyeball : ______________________

Conjunctiva : ________________

Lens : ________________

Vision : ________________

Nose

External noses : ________________

Nostrils : ________________

Nasal septum : ________________

Sinuses ________________

Ear

External ear : ________________

Tympanic membrane : ________________

Hearing acuity : ________________

Mouth

Lips : ________________

Odors : ________________

Teeth : ________________

Tongue : ________________

Speech : ________________

Neck

Thyroid gland and lymph node enlargement:

Inspection : ________________

____

____

Palpation : ________________

____

____

Chest

Inspection : ________________

Palpation : ________________

Percussion : ________________

Auscultation : ________________

Abdomen

Inspection : ________________

Palpation : ________________

Auscultation : ________________________________

Percussion : ________________________________

Genitalia : ________________________________

____

Back : Mention any abnormal posturing: Lordosis/Scoliosis/Kyphosis

Impression : ________________________________

Extremities : Present/Absent/Any illness (specify)

: ________________________________

List of Nursing Diagnosis

1.
2.
3.
4.
5.
6.
7.

Nursing care plan

Assessment of the problems	Nursing diagnosis	Goals/Objectives	Interventions	Implementation	Rationale	Evaluations

Contd...

Contd...

Assessment of the problems	Nursing diagnosis	Goals/Objectives	Interventions	Implementation	Rationale	Evaluations

Contd...

Contd...

Assessment of the problems	Nursing diagnosis	Goals/Objectives	Interventions	Implementation	Rationale	Evaluations

Contd...

Contd...

Assessment of the problems	Nursing diagnosis	Goals/Objectives	Interventions	Implementation	Rationale	Evaluations

Health Education

Recording of Procedure

Sl No.	Date	Name of the beneficiary	Age/Sex	Problem	Procedure done	Remarks/ Finding	Signature of the student

Summary

Conclusion

Signature of the Student
Date:

Signature of the Clinical Instructor
Date:

Family Care Plan

Case 2

Identification Data

House Number: ______________________

Name of the Informer: ______________________

Age: ______________________

Sex: ______________________

Name of Head of the Family: ______________________

Address: ______________________

____

____

____

Type of Family: ______________________

Family Size: ______________________

Religion: ______________________

Caste: ______________________

Educational Status: ______________________

Occupational Status: ______________________

Income of the Family: ₹ ______________________/month

Mother Tongue: ______________________

Student Data

Name of the Student: ______________________

Course: ______________________

Class: ______________________

Date of Care Started: ______________________

Date of Care Ended: ______________________

Family Composition

Sl No.	Name of the family members	Age	Sex	Relationship with head of the family	Education status	Occupation status	Health status
1.							
2.							
3.							
4.							
5.							
6.							
7.							

Socioeconomic Status

Family Tree

Past Medical History

Past Surgical History

Present History of Illness

Housing Pattern (Floor Map)

Housing and Environmental Condition

Type of house	:	
Roof	:	Thatch/Thatti/Tilled/Terraced/Others
Floor	:	Mud/Tiled/Cemented/Others
Wall	:	Thatti/Mud/Brick/Cement plastered/Others
Housing pattern	:	Pucca/Semi-pucca/Kutcha/Others
Possession	:	Own house/Rental house/Leased
Area (square feet)	:	Adequate/Inadequate
Ventilation	:	Natural/Artificial
Number of rooms	:	
Doors/Windows	:	Adequate/Inadequate
Electricity	:	Available/Not available
Mode of lighting	:	Oil lamp/Kerosene/Electric bulb/Others
Water supply	:	Adequate/Inadequate
Mode of water supply	:	Well/Public tap/Hand pump/Others
Latrine	:	Service/Water seal/Open field
Drain	:	Open/Closed/Nil
Street light	:	Yes/No
Street road condition	:	Cement/Tar/Mud/Others
Type of fuel used	:	Firewood/Kerosene/Gas/Cow dung/Biogas
Open space around the house	:	Yes/No
Garden	:	Yes/No
Water stagnation	:	Yes/No
Disposal of waste	:	Drum/Open space/Manure pit/Burning/Throwing into street/Separate
Livestock and poultry	:	Available/Not available
If available	:	Shed/Separate
	:	Attached/Mixed
Healthcare facilities	:	GH/PHC/SC/Private doctors/Others
Medical aid available in the street	:	Doctor/Homeo/Siddha/Village vaidyas/Others
Playground in the street	:	Available/Not available
Social institution	:	Bank/Post office/Police station/Market/Transport
Educational institution	:	Primary school/Secondary school/HSS/College/Night school/Adult school/Crèche
Religious institution	:	Temple/Church/Mosque/Others
Presence of rodents	:	
Presence of stray dog	:	
Presence of domestic animals	:	
Presence of insects	:	

Economical Status

Income : ____________________/month
Source of income : ____________________
Number of earning members : ____________________
Expenditure : ____________________/month
Rent : ____________________/month
Food : ____________________/month
Health : ____________________/month
School : ____________________/month
Miscellaneous : ____________________/month
Own properties : Land/Vehicle/House/Others

Transportation

Bus : ____________________; specify, which bus: ____________________
Auto rickshaw : ____________________ Yes/No
Four wheelers : ____________________ Yes/No
Train : ____________________ Yes/No
Airway : ____________________ Yes/No

Communication

Face to face : ____
Mobile : ____
Telephone : ____
Through letter : ____
Internet : ____

Personal hobbies

Recreational activity : ____

Nutritional Status of Family

Dietary pattern : Vegetarian/Nonvegetarian/Ovo vegetarian
Frequency of nonvegetarian : ____
Food habit: Number of meals : ____/day
Cooking method : ____
Staple food : ____
Sources of food items
(vegetables) : ____
Storage of food items : ____
Usage of processed food items : ____

Beneficiary data

Name of beneficiary : ______________________

Age : ______________________

Sex : ______________________

Menu plan

Sl No.	Type of food	Amount of food	Calories (kcal)
Breakfast			
1.			
2.			
Midmorning			
1.			
2.			
Lunch			
1.			
2.			
3.			
Evening			
1.			
2.			
Dinner			
1.			
2.			
3.			
		Total	

Amount allotted for nutrition : ______________________

Use of:

- Vegetables : ______________________
- Fruits : ______________________
- Cereals/Pulses/Nuts : ______________________

Plan for Home Visit

Sl No.	Name of the beneficiary	Date	Needs/Problems	Preventions	Short-term goals	Long-term goals

Physical Examination

General appearance

Nourishment : ______________________

Body built : ______________________

Health : ______________________

Activity : ______________________

Mental status

Consciousness : ______________________

Look : ______________________

Vital signs

Temperature : ______________________°C

Pulse : ______________________/minute

Respiration : ______________________/minute

Blood pressure : ______________________mm Hg

Anthropometric measurement

Height or length (cm) : ______________________

Weight (kg) : ______________________

Chest circumference (cm) : ______________________

Mid-arm circumference (cm) : ______________________

Body mass index (BMI) : ______________________

Skin condition : ______________________

Color : ______________________

Texture : ______________________

Lesion : ______________________

Sensation : ______________________

Head and face

Scalp : ______________________

Face : ______________________

Hair color : ______________________

Eye

Eyebrows : ______________________

Eyelashes : ______________________

Eyelids : ______________________

Eyeball : ______________________

Conjunctiva : ____________________

Lens : ____________________

Vision : ____________________

Nose

External noses : ____________________

Nostrils : ____________________

Nasal septum : ____________________

Sinuses ____________________

Ear

External ear : ____________________

Tympanic membrane : ____________________

Hearing acuity : ____________________

Mouth

Lips : ____________________

Odors : ____________________

Teeth : ____________________

Tongue : ____________________

Speech : ____________________

Neck

Thyroid gland and lymph node enlargement:

Inspection : ____________________

____

____

Palpation : ____________________

____

____

Chest

Inspection : ____________________

Palpation : ____________________

Percussion : ____________________

Auscultation : ____________________

Abdomen

Inspection : ____________________

Palpation : ____________________

Auscultation : ______________________________

Percussion : ______________________________

Genitalia : ______________________________

____

Back : Mention any abnormal posturing: Lordosis/Scoliosis/Kyphosis

Impression : ______________________________

Extremities : Present/Absent/Any illness (specify)

: ______________________________

List of Nursing Diagnosis

1.
2.
3.
4.
5.
6.
7.

Nursing care plan

Assessment of the problems	Nursing diagnosis	Goals/Objectives	Interventions	Implementation	Rationale	Evaluations

Contd...

Contd...

Assessment of the problems	Nursing diagnosis	Goals/Objectives	Interventions	Implementation	Rationale	Evaluations

Contd...

Contd...

Assessment of the problems	Nursing diagnosis	Goals/Objectives	Interventions	Implementation	Rationale	Evaluations

Contd...

Contd...

Assessment of the problems	Nursing diagnosis	Goals/Objectives	Interventions	Implementation	Rationale	Evaluations

Health Education

Recording of Procedure

Sl No.	Date	Name of the beneficiary	Age/Sex	Problem	Procedure done	Remarks/ Finding	Signature of the student

Summary

Conclusion

Signature of the Student
Date:

Signature of the Clinical Instructor
Date:

Family Care Plan

Case 3

Identification Data

House Number: ______________________

Name of the Informer: ______________________

Age: ______________________

Sex: ______________________

Name of Head of the Family: ______________________

Address: ______________________

____

____

____

Type of Family: ______________________

Family Size: ______________________

Religion: ______________________

Caste: ______________________

Educational Status: ______________________

Occupational Status: ______________________

Income of the Family: ₹ ______________________/month

Mother Tongue: ______________________

Student Data

Name of the Student: ______________________

Course: ______________________

Class: ______________________

Date of Care Started: ______________________

Date of Care Ended: ______________________

Family Composition

Sl No.	Name of the family members	Age	Sex	Relationship with head of the family	Education status	Occupation status	Health status
1.							
2.							
3.							
4.							
5.							
6.							
7.							

Socioeconomic Status

Family Tree

Past Medical History

Past Surgical History

Present History of Illness

Housing Pattern (Floor Map)

Housing and Environmental Condition

Type of house	:
Roof	: Thatch/Thatti/Tilled/Terraced/Others
Floor	: Mud/Tiled/Cemented/Others
Wall	: Thatti/Mud/Brick/Cement plastered/Others
Housing pattern	: Pucca/Semi-pucca/Kutcha/Others
Possession	: Own house/Rental house/Leased
Area (square feet)	: Adequate/Inadequate
Ventilation	: Natural/Artificial
Number of rooms	:
Doors/Windows	: Adequate/Inadequate
Electricity	: Available/Not available
Mode of lighting	: Oil lamp/Kerosene/Electric bulb/Others
Water supply	: Adequate/Inadequate
Mode of water supply	: Well/Public tap/Hand pump/Others
Latrine	: Service/Water seal/Open field
Drain	: Open/Closed/Nil
Street light	: Yes/No
Street road condition	: Cement/Tar/Mud/Others
Type of fuel used	: Firewood/Kerosene/Gas/Cow dung/Biogas
Open space around the house	: Yes/No
Garden	: Yes/No
Water stagnation	: Yes/No
Disposal of waste	: Drum/Open space/Manure pit/Burning/Throwing into street/Separate
Livestock and poultry	: Available/Not available
If available	: Shed/Separate
	: Attached/Mixed
Healthcare facilities	: GH/PHC/SC/Private doctors/Others
Medical aid available in the street	: Doctor/Homeo/Siddha/Village vaidyas/Others
Playground in the street	: Available/Not available
Social institution	: Bank/Post office/Police station/Market/Transport
Educational institution	: Primary school/Secondary school/HSS/College/Night school/Adult school/Crèche
Religious institution	: Temple/Church/Mosque/Others
Presence of rodents	:
Presence of stray dog	:
Presence of domestic animals	:
Presence of insects	:

Economical Status

Income : ____________________/month
Source of income : ____________________
Number of earning members : ____________________
Expenditure : ____________________/month
Rent : ____________________/month
Food : ____________________/month
Health : ____________________/month
School : ____________________/month
Miscellaneous : ____________________/month
Own properties : Land/Vehicle/House/Others

Transportation

Bus : ____________________; specify, which bus: ____________________
Auto rickshaw : ____________________ Yes/No
Four wheelers : ____________________ Yes/No
Train : ____________________ Yes/No
Airway : ____________________ Yes/No

Communication

Face to face : ____________________
Mobile : ____________________
Telephone : ____________________
Through letter : ____________________
Internet : ____________________

Personal hobbies

Recreational activity : ____________________

Nutritional Status of Family

Dietary pattern : Vegetarian/Nonvegetarian/Ovo vegetarian
Frequency of nonvegetarian : ____________________
Food habit: Number of meals : ____________________/day
Cooking method : ____________________
Staple food : ____________________
Sources of food items
(vegetables) : ____________________
Storage of food items : ____________________
Usage of processed food items : ____________________

Beneficiary data

Name of beneficiary : ____________________

Age : ____________________

Sex : ____________________

Menu plan

Sl No.	Type of food	Amount of food	Calories (kcal)
Breakfast			
1.			
2.			
Midmorning			
1.			
2.			
Lunch			
1.			
2.			
3.			
Evening			
1.			
2.			
Dinner			
1.			
2.			
3.			
		Total	

Amount allotted for nutrition : ____________________

Use of:

- Vegetables : ____________________
- Fruits : ____________________
- Cereals/Pulses/Nuts : ____________________

Plan for Home Visit

Sl No.	Name of the beneficiary	Date	Needs/Problems	Preventions	Short-term goals	Long-term goals

Physical Examination

General appearance

Nourishment : ____________________

Body built : ____________________

Health : ____________________

Activity : ____________________

Mental status

Consciousness : ____________________

Look : ____________________

Vital signs

Temperature : ____________________°C

Pulse : ____________________/minute

Respiration : ____________________/minute

Blood pressure : ____________________mm Hg

Anthropometric measurement

Height or length (cm) : ____________________

Weight (kg) : ____________________

Chest circumference (cm) : ____________________

Mid-arm circumference (cm) : ____________________

Body mass index (BMI) : ____________________

Skin condition : ____________________

Color : ____________________

Texture : ____________________

Lesion : ____________________

Sensation : ____________________

Head and face

Scalp : ____________________

Face : ____________________

Hair color : ____________________

Eye

Eyebrows : ____________________

Eyelashes : ____________________

Eyelids : ____________________

Eyeball : ____________________

Conjunctiva : ____________________
Lens : ____________________
Vision : ____________________

Nose

External noses : ____________________
Nostrils : ____________________
Nasal septum : ____________________
Sinuses ____________________

Ear

External ear : ____________________
Tympanic membrane : ____________________
Hearing acuity : ____________________

Mouth

Lips : ____________________
Odors : ____________________
Teeth : ____________________
Tongue : ____________________
Speech : ____________________

Neck

Thyroid gland and lymph node enlargement:

Inspection : ____________________
____
____

Palpation : ____________________
____
____

Chest

Inspection : ____________________
Palpation : ____________________
Percussion : ____________________
Auscultation : ____________________

Abdomen

Inspection : ____________________
Palpation : ____________________

Auscultation : ____________________

Percussion : ____________________

Genitalia : ____________________

____

Back : Mention any abnormal posturing: Lordosis/Scoliosis/Kyphosis

Impression : ____________________

Extremities : Present/Absent/Any illness (specify)

: ____________________

List of Nursing Diagnosis

1.
2.
3.
4.
5.
6.
7.

Nursing care plan

Assessment of the problems	Nursing diagnosis	Goals/Objectives	Interventions	Implementation	Rationale	Evaluations

Contd...

Contd...

Assessment of the problems	Nursing diagnosis	Goals/Objectives	Interventions	Implementation	Rationale	Evaluations

Contd...

Contd...

Assessment of the problems	Nursing diagnosis	Goals/Objectives	Interventions	Implementation	Rationale	Evaluations

Contd...

Contd...

Assessment of the problems	Nursing diagnosis	Goals/Objectives	Interventions	Implementation	Rationale	Evaluations

Health Education

Recording of Procedure

Sl No.	Date	Name of the beneficiary	Age/Sex	Problem	Procedure done	Remarks/ Finding	Signature of the student

Summary

Conclusion

Signature of the Student
Date:

Signature of the Clinical Instructor
Date:

Family Care Study

Case 1

Identification Data

House Number: ____________________

Name of the Informer: ____________________

Age: ____________________

Sex: ____________________

Name of Head of the Family: ____________________

Address: ____________________

____

____

____

Type of Family: ____________________

Family Size: ____________________

Religion: ____________________

Caste: ____________________

Educational Status: ____________________

Occupational Status: ____________________

Income of the Family: ₹ ____________________/month

Mother Tongue: ____________________

Student Data

Name of the Student: ____________________

Course: ____________________

Class: ____________________

Date of Care Started: ____________________

Date of Care Ended: ____________________

Family Composition

Sl No.	Name of the family members	Age	Sex	Relationship with head of the family	Education status	Occupation status	Health status
1.							
2.							
3.							
4.							
5.							
6.							
7.							

Socioeconomic Status

Family Tree

Past Medical History

Past Surgical History

Present History of Illness

Housing Pattern (Floor Map)

Housing and Environmental Condition

Type of house	:
Roof	: Thatch/Thatti/Tilled/Terraced/Others
Floor	: Mud/Tiled/Cemented/Others
Wall	: Thatti/Mud/Brick/Cement plastered/Others
Housing pattern	: Pucca/Semi-pucca/Kutcha/Others
Possession	: Own house/Rental house/Leased
Area (square feet)	: Adequate/Inadequate
Ventilation	: Natural/Artificial
Number of rooms	:
Doors/Windows	: Adequate/Inadequate
Electricity	: Available/Not available
Mode of lighting	: Oil lamp/Kerosene/Electric bulb/Others
Water supply	: Adequate/Inadequate
Mode of water supply	: Well/Public tap/Hand pump/Others
Latrine	: Service/Water seal/Open field
Drain	: Open/Closed/Nil
Street light	: Yes/No
Street road condition	: Cement/Tar/Mud/Others
Type of fuel used	: Firewood/Kerosene/Gas/Cow dung/Biogas
Open space around the house	: Yes/No
Garden	: Yes/No
Water stagnation	: Yes/No
Disposal of waste	: Drum/Open space/Manure pit/Burning/Throwing into street/Separate
Livestock and poultry	: Available/Not available
If available	: Shed/Separate
	: Attached/Mixed
Healthcare facilities	: GH/PHC/SC/Private doctors/Others
Medical aid available in the street	: Doctor/Homeo/Siddha/Village vaidyas/Others
Playground in the street	: Available/Not available
Social institution	: Bank/Post office/Police station/Market/Transport
Educational institution	: Primary school/Secondary school/HSS/College/Night school/Adult school/Crèche
Religious institution	: Temple/Church/Mosque/Others
Presence of rodents	:
Presence of stray dog	:
Presence of domestic animals	:
Presence of insects	:

Economical Status

Income : ______________________/month
Source of income : ______________________
Number of earning members : ______________________
Expenditure : ______________________/month
Rent : ______________________/month
Food : ______________________/month
Health : ______________________/month
School : ______________________/month
Miscellaneous : ______________________/month
Own properties : Land/Vehicle/House/Others

Transportation

Bus : ______________________; specify, which bus: ______________________
Auto rickshaw : ______________________ Yes/No
Four wheelers : ______________________ Yes/No
Train : ______________________ Yes/No
Airway : ______________________ Yes/No

Communication

Face to face : ______________________
Mobile : ______________________
Telephone : ______________________
Through letter : ______________________
Internet : ______________________

Personal hobbies

Recreational activity : ______________________

Nutritional Status of Family

Dietary pattern : Vegetarian/Nonvegetarian/Ovo vegetarian
Frequency of nonvegetarian : ______________________
Food habit: Number of meals : ______________________/day
Cooking method : ______________________
Staple food : ______________________
Sources of food items (vegetables) : ______________________
Storage of food items : ______________________
Usage of processed food items : ______________________

Beneficiary data

Name of beneficiary : ______________________

Age : ______________________

Sex : ______________________

Menu plan

Sl No.	Types of food	Amount of food	Calories (kcal)
Breakfast			
1.			
2.			
Midmorning			
1.			
2.			
Lunch			
1.			
2.			
3.			
Evening			
1.			
2.			
Dinner			
1.			
2.			
3.			
		Total	

Amount allotted for nutrition : ______________________

Use of:

- Vegetables : ______________________
- Fruits : ______________________
- Cereals/Pulses/Nuts : ______________________

Cooking demonstration

____

____

____

____

____

____

Plan for Home Visit

Sl No.	Name of the beneficiary	Date	Needs/Problems	Prevention	Short-term goal	Long-term goal

Physical Examination

General appearance

Nourishment : ______

Body built : ______

Health : ______

Activity : ______

Mental status

Consciousness : ______

Look : ______

Vital signs

Temperature : ______°C

Pulse : ______/minute

Respiration : ______/minute

Blood pressure : ______mm Hg

Anthropometric measurement

Height or length (cm) : ______

Weight (kg) : ______

Chest circumference (cm) : ______

Mid-arm circumference (cm) : ______________________

Body mass index (BMI) : ______________________

Skin condition : ______________________

Color : ______________________

Texture : ______________________

Lesion : ______________________

Sensation : ______________________

Head and face

Scalp : ______________________

Face : ______________________

Hair color : ______________________

Eye

Eyebrows : ______________________

Eyelashes : ______________________

Eyelids : ______________________

Eyeball : ______________________

Conjunctiva : ______________________

Lens : ______________________

Vision : ______________________

Nose

External noses : ______________________

Nostrils : ______________________

Nasal septum : ______________________

Sinuses ______________________

Ear

External ear : ______________________

Tympanic membrane : ______________________

Hearing acuity : ______________________

Mouth

Lips : ______________________

Odors : ______________________

Teeth : ______________________

Tongue : ______________________

Speech : ______________________

Neck

Thyroid gland and lymph node enlargement:

Inspection : ____________________

Palpation : ____________________

Chest

Inspection : ____________________

Palpation : ____________________

Percussion : ____________________

Auscultation : ____________________

Abdomen

Inspection : ____________________

Palpation : ____________________

Auscultation : ____________________

Percussion : ____________________

Genitalia

: ____________________

Back : Mention any abnormal posturing: Lordosis/Scoliosis/Kyphosis

Impression : ____________________

Extremities : Present/Absent/Any illness (specify)

: ____________________

Investigation

Sl No.	Investigation	Normal value	Patient value	Remarks

Medication

Sl No.	Medication	Route/Amount	Action	Side effect	Remarks

List of Nursing Diagnosis

1.
2.
3.
4.
5.
6.
7.

Book Picture

Nursing Diagnosis

1.
2.
3.
4.
5.
6.
7.

Nursing care plan

Assessment of the problems	Nursing diagnosis	Goals/Objectives	Interventions	Implementation	Rationale	Evaluations

Contd...

Contd...

Assessment of the problems	Nursing diagnosis	Goals/Objectives	Interventions	Implementation	Rationale	Evaluations

Contd...

Contd...

Assessment of the problems	Nursing diagnosis	Goals/Objectives	Interventions	Implementation	Rationale	Evaluations

Contd...

Contd...

Assessment of the problems	Nursing diagnosis	Goals/Objectives	Interventions	Implementation	Rationale	Evaluations

Contd...

Contd...

Assessment of the problems	Nursing diagnosis	Goals/Objectives	Interventions	Implementation	Rationale	Evaluations

Health Education

Recording of Procedure

Sl No.	Date	Name of the beneficiary	Age/Sex	Problem	Procedure done	Remarks/ Findings	Signature of the student

Summary

Conclusion

Bibliography

Signature of the Student
Date:

Signature of the Clinical Instructor
Date:

Family Care Study

Case 2

Identification Data

House Number: ______

Name of the Informer: ______

Age: ______

Sex: ______

Name of Head of the Family: ______

Address: ______

______

______

______

Type of Family: ______

Family Size: ______

Religion: ______

Caste: ______

Educational Status: ______

Occupational Status: ______

Income of the Family: ₹ ______/month

Mother Tongue: ______

Student Data

Name of the Student: ______

Course: ______

Class: ______

Date of Care Started: ______

Date of Care Ended: ______

Family Composition

Sl No.	Name of the family members	Age	Sex	Relationship with head of the family	Education status	Occupation status	Health status
1.							
2.							
3.							
4.							
5.							
6.							
7.							

Socioeconomic Status

Family Tree

Past Medical History

Past Surgical History

Present History of Illness

Housing Pattern (Floor Map)

Housing and Environmental Condition

Type of house	:
Roof	: Thatch/Thatti/Tilled/Terraced/Others
Floor	: Mud/Tiled/Cemented/Others
Wall	: Thatti/Mud/Brick/Cement plastered/Others
Housing pattern	: Pucca/Semi-pucca/Kutcha/Others
Possession	: Own house/Rental house/Leased
Area (square feet)	: Adequate/Inadequate
Ventilation	: Natural/Artificial
Number of rooms	:
Doors/Windows	: Adequate/Inadequate
Electricity	: Available/Not available
Mode of lighting	: Oil lamp/Kerosene/Electric bulb/Others
Water supply	: Adequate/Inadequate
Mode of water supply	: Well/Public tap/Hand pump/Others
Latrine	: Service/Water seal/Open field
Drain	: Open/Closed/Nil
Street light	: Yes/No
Street road condition	: Cement/Tar/Mud/Others
Type of fuel used	: Firewood/Kerosene/Gas/Cow dung/Biogas
Open space around the house	: Yes/No
Garden	: Yes/No
Water stagnation	: Yes/No
Disposal of waste	: Drum/Open space/Manure pit/Burning/Throwing into street/Separate
Livestock and poultry	: Available/Not available
If available	: Shed/Separate
	: Attached/Mixed
Healthcare facilities	: GH/PHC/SC/Private doctors/Others
Medical aid available in the street	: Doctor/Homeo/Siddha/Village vaidyas/Others
Playground in the street	: Available/Not available
Social institution	: Bank/Post office/Police station/Market/Transport
Educational institution	: Primary school/Secondary school/HSS/College/Night school/Adult school/Crèche
Religious institution	: Temple/Church/Mosque/Others
Presence of rodents	:
Presence of stray dog	:
Presence of domestic animals	:
Presence of insects	:

Economical Status

Income : ____________________/month

Source of income : ____________________

Number of earning members : ____________________

Expenditure : ____________________/month

Rent : ____________________/month

Food : ____________________/month

Health : ____________________/month

School : ____________________/month

Miscellaneous : ____________________/month

Own properties : Land/Vehicle/House/Others

Transportation

Bus : ____________________; specify, which bus: ____________________

Auto rickshaw : ____________________ Yes/No

Four wheelers : ____________________ Yes/No

Train : ____________________ Yes/No

Airway : ____________________ Yes/No

Communication

Face to face : ____

Mobile : ____

Telephone : ____

Through letter : ____

Internet : ____

Personal hobbies

Recreational activity : ____

Nutritional Status of Family

Dietary pattern : Vegetarian/Nonvegetarian/Ovo vegetarian

Frequency of nonvegetarian : ____

Food habit: Number of meals : ____/day

Cooking method : ____

Staple food : ____

Sources of food items

(vegetables) : ____

Storage of food items : ____

Usage of processed food items : ____

Beneficiary data

Name of beneficiary : ____________________

Age : ____________________

Sex : ____________________

Menu plan

Sl No.	Types of food	Amount of food	Calories (kcal)
Breakfast			
1.			
2.			
Midmorning			
1.			
2.			
Lunch			
1.			
2.			
3.			
Evening			
1.			
2.			
Dinner			
1.			
2.			
3.			
		Total	

Amount allotted for nutrition : ____________________

Use of:

- Vegetables : ____________________
- Fruits : ____________________
- Cereals/Pulses/Nuts : ____________________

Cooking demonstration

____

____

____

____

____

____

Plan for Home Visit

Sl No.	Name of the beneficiary	Date	Needs/Problems	Prevention	Short-term goal	Long-term goal

Physical Examination

General appearance

Nourishment : ____________________

Body built : ____________________

Health : ____________________

Activity : ____________________

Mental status

Consciousness : ____________________

Look : ____________________

Vital signs

Temperature : ____________________°C

Pulse : ____________________/minute

Respiration : ____________________/minute

Blood pressure : ____________________mm Hg

Anthropometric measurement

Height or length (cm) : ____________________

Weight (kg) : ____________________

Chest circumference (cm) : ____________________

Mid-arm circumference (cm) : ____________________

Body mass index (BMI) : ____________________

Skin condition : ____________________

Color : ____________________

Texture : ____________________

Lesion : ____________________

Sensation : ____________________

Head and face

Scalp : ____________________

Face : ____________________

Hair color : ____________________

Eye

Eyebrows : ____________________

Eyelashes : ____________________

Eyelids : ____________________

Eyeball : ____________________

Conjunctiva : ____________________

Lens : ____________________

Vision : ____________________

Nose

External noses : ____________________

Nostrils : ____________________

Nasal septum : ____________________

Sinuses ____________________

Ear

External ear : ____________________

Tympanic membrane : ____________________

Hearing acuity : ____________________

Mouth

Lips : ____________________

Odors : ____________________

Teeth : ____________________

Tongue : ____________________

Speech : ____________________

Neck

Thyroid gland and lymph node enlargement:

Inspection : ____________________

____

____

Palpation : ____________________

____

____

Chest

Inspection : ____________________

Palpation : ____________________

Percussion : ____________________

Auscultation : ____________________

Abdomen

Inspection : ____________________

Palpation : ____________________

Auscultation : ____________________

Percussion : ____________________

Genitalia

: ____________________

____

Back : Mention any abnormal posturing: Lordosis/Scoliosis/Kyphosis

Impression : ____________________

Extremities : Present/Absent/Any illness (specify)

: ____________________

Investigation

Sl No.	Investigation	Normal value	Patient value	Remarks

Medication

Sl No.	Medication	Route/Amount	Action	Side effect	Remarks

List of Nursing Diagnosis

1.
2.
3.
4.
5.
6.
7.

Book Picture

Nursing Diagnosis

1.
2.
3.
4.
5.
6.
7.

Nursing care plan

Assessment of the problems	Nursing diagnosis	Goals/Objectives	Interventions	Implementation	Rationale	Evaluations

Contd...

Contd...

Assessment of the problems	Nursing diagnosis	Goals/Objectives	Interventions	Implementation	Rationale	Evaluations

Contd...

Contd...

Assessment of the problems	Nursing diagnosis	Goals/Objectives	Interventions	Implementation	Rationale	Evaluations

Contd...

Contd...

Assessment of the problems	Nursing diagnosis	Goals/Objectives	Interventions	Implementation	Rationale	Evaluations

Contd...

Contd...

Assessment of the problems	Nursing diagnosis	Goals/Objectives	Interventions	Implementation	Rationale	Evaluations

Health Education

Recording of Procedure

Sl No.	Date	Name of the beneficiary	Age/Sex	Problem	Procedure done	Remarks/ Findings	Signature of the student

Summary

Conclusion

Bibliography

Signature of the Student
Date:

Signature of the Clinical Instructor
Date:

Antenatal Clinic

Introduction

Objectives

Purpose

Functions

Sl No.	Name of the mother	Age	Date of examination	Obstetrical score	LMP*	EDD†	Weeks	Fundal weight	Presentation	Position	Engagement	Hb%	FHR‡	Weight of the mother	Remarks
1.															
2.															
3.															
4.															
5.															
6.															
7.															
8.															
9.															

Contd...

Contd...

Sl No.	Name of the mother	Age	Date of examination	Obstetrical score	LMP*	EDD†	Weeks	Fundal weight	Presentation	Position	Engagement	Hb%	FHR‡	Weight of the mother	Remarks
10.															
11.															
12.															
13.															
14.															
15.															
16.															
17.															
18.															

*LMP, last menstrual period; †EDD, expected date of delivery; ‡FHR, fetal heart rate.

Summary

Conclusion

Signature of the Student
Date:

Signature of the Clinical Instructor
Date:

Postnatal Clinic

Introduction

General Objectives

Purpose

Functions

Sl No.	Name of the mother	Age	Obstetrical score	Date of delivery	Weight of mother (kg)	Sex of the baby	Height of the baby	Weight of the baby	Health status of mother and baby	Health status of baby after vaccination	Remarks
1.											
2.											
3.											
4.											
5.											
6.											
7.											
8.											

Contd...

Contd...

Sl No.	Name of the mother	Age	Obstetrical score	Date of delivery	Weight of mother (kg)	Sex of the baby	Height of the baby	Weight of the baby	Health status of mother and baby	Health status of baby after vaccination	Remarks
9.											
10.											
11.											
12.											
13.											
14.											
15.											
16.											
17.											

Summary

Conclusion

Signature of the Student
Date:

Signature of the Clinical Instructor
Date:

Under-five Clinic

Introduction

Objectives

Purpose

Functions

Immunization Schedule

Sl No.	Age	Vaccine	Given on	Remarks
1.				
2.				
3.				
4.				

Contd...

Contd...

Sl No.	Age	Vaccine	Given on	Remarks
5.				
6.				
7.				
8.				
9.				
10.				

Conclusion

Family Welfare Clinic

Introduction

Report

Sl No.	Name of the mother	Age	Height	Weight	Vital signs	Health status	Obstetrical score	Number of living child	Method of family planning
1.									
2.									
3.									
4.									
5.									
6.									
7.									
8.									
9.									
10.									
11.									
12.									
13.									
14.									
15.									
16.									
17.									
18.									

Antenatal Assessment

Case 1

Card Number ____________________

Mother Profile

Name of the Mother : ____________________
Age of the Mother : ____________________
Age of the Husband : ____________________
Education of the Mother : ____________________
Education of the Husband : ____________________
Occupation of the Mother : ____________________
Occupation of the Husband : ____________________
Family Income Status : ____________________/month
Type of Family : ____________________
Socioeconomic Status : ____________________
Date of Last Antenatal Visit : ____________________
Name of the Doctor : ____________________
Name of the Primary Health Center : ____________________
Address : ____________________
____
____
____

Obstetrical Score : G ______ P ______ A ______ L ______ D ______ S ______
Age at Marriage : ____________________
Use of Contraceptives : ____________________
Relationship with Spouse : Consanguineous/Nonconsanguineous
Diagnosis, if any : ____________________

Family History

Type of family : ____________________
Congenital deformities : Present/Absent
Hereditary disease : Present/Absent

If present means mention : ____________________

____

____

Multiple pregnancies : ____________________

Menstrual History

Age at menarche : ____________________

Duration of menstrual cycles : ____________________

Menstrual cycle regularity : ____________________

Dysmenorrhea/Leukorrhea/

Menorrhagia : ____________________

____

Duration : ____________________

Last menstrual period : Date: __________ Month: __________

Present Obstetrical History

Period of gestational weeks : ____________________

Date of confirmation of pregnancy : ____________________

Last menstrual period : ____________________

Expected date of delivery : ____________________

Quickening : ____________________

Gravida : ____________________

Para : ____________________

Investigation

Sl No.	Investigation	Result

Minor disorders : ____________________

____

____

If any, specify : ______________________________

____

____

Antenatal Examination

Parameters	1st month	2nd month	3rd month	4th month	5th month	6th month	7th month	8th month	9th month
Weight (kg)									
Weight increase (kg)									
Height (cm)									
Temperature									
Pulse									
Respiration									
Blood pressure									

Urine Test

Sugar : ______________________________

Albumin : ______________________________

Inspection

General appearance : ______________________________

Stature (normal/short) : ______________________________

Palpation

Fundal : ______________________________

Abdominal girth : ______________________________

Lateral : ______________________________

Pelvic : ______________________________

Auscultation

Fetal heart rate (FHR) : ______________________________ Regular/Irregular

Past Obstetrical History

Year of last childbirth : ___________________________

Number of children : ___________________________

1	2	3	4

Type of delivery:
- Normal delivery (N)
- Cesarean section (CS)

1	2	3	4

Sex of the child:
- Male (M)
- Female (F)

1	2	3	4

Location : ___________________________

Any complaints after delivery : ___________________________

Sl No.	Age of the child	Type of delivery	Baby alive/dead	Sex of the baby	Birth weight of the baby	Any congenital deformities	Term	Abortion	Remarks
1.									
2.									
3.									
4.									
5.									

Physical Examination

Nourishment : ____________________

Body built : ____________________

Weight : ____________________kg

Height : ____________________cm

Vital signs

Temperature : ____________________

Pulse : ____________________

Respiration : ____________________

Blood pressure : ____________________

Mental status

Consciousness : ____________________

Look : ____________________

Head to Foot Examination

Skin turgor : ____________________

Moisture : ____________________

Warmth/Temperature : ____________________

Face : ____________________

Facial puffiness : ____________________

Lips : ____________________

Eyes : ____________________

Periorbital edema : ____________________

Conjunctiva : Pallor

Mouth : ____________________

Tongue : ____________________

Breast

Inspection : ____________________

____

____

Palpation : ____________________

____

____

Nipples : ____________________

____

____

Abdomen:

Inspection

Size : ____________________

Shape : ____________________

Contour : ____________________

Marks : ____________________

Umbilicus : ____________________

Fetal movements : ____________________

Skin changes : ____________________

Contractions : Present/Absent

Palpation

Fundal : Description

Inference : ____________________

Lic : ____________________

Presentation : ____________________

Lateral

Left side : Description

Right side : Description inference: Position

Pelvic

First pelvic grip : ____________________

Second pelvic grip : ____________________

Inference

Position : ____________________

Engagement/Not engagement : ____________________

Attitude : ____________________

Pawlik's grip : Fixed/Mobile

Auscultation

Fetal heart rate (FHR) : ____________________

Rhythm : ____________________

Location : ____________________

Extremities

Ankle edema : ____________________

Capillary refill : ____________________

Cyanosis : ____________________

Palm fas delivery : ____________________

Health Education

Summary

Conclusion

Signature of the Student
Date:

Signature of the Clinical Coordinator
Date:

Antenatal Assessment

Case 2

Card Number ____________________

Mother Profile

Name of the Mother : ____________________

Age of the Mother : ____________________

Age of the Husband : ____________________

Education of the Mother : ____________________

Education of the Husband : ____________________

Occupation of the Mother : ____________________

Occupation of the Husband : ____________________

Family Income Status : ____________________/month

Type of Family : ____________________

Socioeconomic Status : ____________________

Date of Last Antenatal Visit : ____________________

Name of the Doctor : ____________________

Name of the Primary Health Center : ____________________

Address : ____________________

____

____

____

Obstetrical Score : G ______ P ______ A ______ L ______ D ______ S ______

Age at Marriage : ____________________

Use of Contraceptives : ____________________

Relationship with Spouse : Consanguineous/Nonconsanguineous

Diagnosis, if any : ____________________

Family History

Type of family : ____________________

Congenital deformities : Present/Absent

Hereditary disease : Present/Absent

If present means mention : ____________________

____

____

Multiple pregnancies : ____________________

Menstrual History

Age at menarche : ____________________

Duration of menstrual cycles : ____________________

Menstrual cycle regularity : ____________________

Dysmenorrhea/Leukorrhea/
Menorrhagia : ____________________

____

Duration : ____________________

Last menstrual period : Date: __________ Month: __________

Present Obstetrical History

Period of gestational weeks : ____________________

Date of confirmation of pregnancy : ____________________

Last menstrual period : ____________________

Expected date of delivery : ____________________

Quickening : ____________________

Gravida : ____________________

Para : ____________________

Investigation

Sl No.	Investigation	Result

Minor disorders : ____________________

____

____

If any, specify : ________________________________

____

____

Antenatal Examination

Parameters	1st month	2nd month	3rd month	4th month	5th month	6th month	7th month	8th month	9th month
Weight (kg)									
Weight increase (kg)									
Height (cm)									
Temperature									
Pulse									
Respiration									
Blood pressure									

Urine Test

Sugar : ________________________________

Albumin : ________________________________

Inspection

General appearance : ________________________________

Stature (normal/short) : ________________________________

Palpation

Fundal : ________________________________

Abdominal girth : ________________________________

Lateral : ________________________________

Pelvic : ________________________________

Auscultation

Fetal heart rate (FHR) : ________________________ Regular/Irregular

Past Obstetrical History

Year of last childbirth : ______________________

Number of children : ______________________

1	2	3	4

Type of delivery:
- Normal delivery (N)
- Cesarean section (CS)

1	2	3	4

Sex of the child:
- Male (M)
- Female (F)

1	2	3	4

Location : ______________________

Any complaints after delivery : ______________________

Sl No.	Age of the child	Type of delivery	Baby alive/dead	Sex of the baby	Birth weight of the baby	Any congenital deformities	Term	Abortion	Remarks
1.									
2.									
3.									
4.									
5.									

Physical Examination

Nourishment : ____________________

Body built : ____________________

Weight : ____________________kg

Height : ____________________cm

Vital signs

Temperature : ____________________

Pulse : ____________________

Respiration : ____________________

Blood pressure : ____________________

Mental status

Consciousness : ____________________

Look : ____________________

Head to Foot Examination

Skin turgor : ____________________

Moisture : ____________________

Warmth/Temperature : ____________________

Face : ____________________

Facial puffiness : ____________________

Lips : ____________________

Eyes : ____________________

Periorbital edema : ____________________

Conjunctiva : Pallor

Mouth : ____________________

Tongue : ____________________

Breast

Inspection : ____________________

____

____

Palpation : ____________________

____

____

Nipples : ____________________
____
____

Abdomen:

Inspection

Size : ____________________

Shape : ____________________

Contour : ____________________

Marks : ____________________

Umbilicus : ____________________

Fetal movements : ____________________

Skin changes : ____________________

Contractions : Present/Absent

Palpation

Fundal : Description

Inference : ____________________

Lic : ____________________

Presentation : ____________________

Lateral

Left side : Description

Right side : Description inference: Position

Pelvic

First pelvic grip : ____________________

Second pelvic grip : ____________________

Inference

Position : ____________________

Engagement/Not engagement : ____________________

Attitude : ____________________

Pawlik's grip : Fixed/Mobile

Auscultation

Fetal heart rate (FHR) : ____________________

Rhythm : ____________________

Location : ____________________

Extremities

Ankle edema : ____________________

Capillary refill : ____________________

Cyanosis : ____________________

Palm fas delivery : ____________________

Health Education

Summary

Conclusion

Signature of the Student
Date:

Signature of the Clinical Coordinator
Date:

Antenatal Assessment

Case 3

Card Number ______________________

Mother Profile

Name of the Mother : ______________________
Age of the Mother : ______________________
Age of the Husband : ______________________
Education of the Mother : ______________________
Education of the Husband : ______________________
Occupation of the Mother : ______________________
Occupation of the Husband : ______________________
Family Income Status : ______________________/month
Type of Family : ______________________
Socioeconomic Status : ______________________
Date of Last Antenatal Visit : ______________________
Name of the Doctor : ______________________
Name of the Primary Health Center : ______________________
Address : ______________________
____
____
____

Obstetrical Score : G ______ P ______ A ______ L ______ D ______ S ______
Age at Marriage : ______________________
Use of Contraceptives : ______________________
Relationship with Spouse : Consanguineous/Nonconsanguineous
Diagnosis, if any : ______________________

Family History

Type of family : ______________________
Congenital deformities : Present/Absent
Hereditary disease : Present/Absent

If present means mention : ______________________

____

____

Multiple pregnancies : ______________________

Menstrual History

Age at menarche : ______________________

Duration of menstrual cycles : ______________________

Menstrual cycle regularity : ______________________

Dysmenorrhea/Leukorrhea/
Menorrhagia : ______________________

____

Duration : ______________________

Last menstrual period : Date: ____________ Month: ____________

Present Obstetrical History

Period of gestational weeks : ______________________

Date of confirmation of pregnancy : ______________________

Last menstrual period : ______________________

Expected date of delivery : ______________________

Quickening : ______________________

Gravida : ______________________

Para : ______________________

Investigation

Sl No.	Investigation	Result

Minor disorders : ______________________

____

____

If any, specify : ______________________________

____

____

Antenatal Examination

Parameters	1st month	2nd month	3rd month	4th month	5th month	6th month	7th month	8th month	9th month
Weight (kg)									
Weight increase (kg)									
Height (cm)									
Temperature									
Pulse									
Respiration									
Blood pressure									

Urine Test

Sugar : ______________________________

Albumin : ______________________________

Inspection

General appearance : ______________________________

Stature (normal/short) : ______________________________

Palpation

Fundal : ______________________________

Abdominal girth : ______________________________

Lateral : ______________________________

Pelvic : ______________________________

Auscultation

Fetal heart rate (FHR) : ______________________________ Regular/Irregular

Past Obstetrical History

Year of last childbirth : ____________________

Number of children : ____________________

1	2	3	4

Type of delivery:

- Normal delivery (N)
- Cesarean section (CS)

1	2	3	4

Sex of the child:

- Male (M)
- Female (F)

1	2	3	4

Location : ____________________

Any complaints after delivery : ____________________

Sl No.	Age of the child	Type of delivery	Baby alive/dead	Sex of the baby	Birth weight of the baby	Any congenital deformities	Term	Abortion	Remarks
1.									
2.									
3.									
4.									
5.									

Physical Examination

Nourishment : ____________________

Body built : ____________________

Weight : ____________________ kg

Height : ____________________ cm

Vital signs

Temperature : ____________________

Pulse : ____________________

Respiration : ____________________

Blood pressure : ____________________

Mental status

Consciousness : ____________________

Look : ____________________

Head to Foot Examination

Skin turgor : ____________________

Moisture : ____________________

Warmth/Temperature : ____________________

Face : ____________________

Facial puffiness : ____________________

Lips : ____________________

Eyes : ____________________

Periorbital edema : ____________________

Conjunctiva : Pallor

Mouth : ____________________

Tongue : ____________________

Breast

Inspection : ____________________

____

____

Palpation : ____________________

____

____

Nipples : ______________________________
____
____

Abdomen:

Inspection

Size : ______________________________

Shape : ______________________________

Contour : ______________________________

Marks : ______________________________

Umbilicus : ______________________________

Fetal movements : ______________________________

Skin changes : ______________________________

Contractions : Present/Absent

Palpation

Fundal : Description

Inference : ______________________________

Lic : ______________________________

Presentation : ______________________________

Lateral

Left side : Description

Right side : Description inference: Position

Pelvic

First pelvic grip : ______________________________

Second pelvic grip : ______________________________

Inference

Position : ______________________________

Engagement/Not engagement : ______________________________

Attitude : ______________________________

Pawlik's grip : Fixed/Mobile

Auscultation

Fetal heart rate (FHR) : ______________________________

Rhythm : ______________________________

Location : ______________________________

Extremities

Ankle edema : ________________

Capillary refill : ________________

Cyanosis : ________________

Palm fas delivery : ________________

Health Education

Summary

Conclusion

Signature of the Student
Date:

Signature of the Clinical Coordinator
Date:

Antenatal Assessment

Case 4

Card Number ______________________

Mother Profile

Name of the Mother : ______________________
Age of the Mother : ______________________
Age of the Husband : ______________________
Education of the Mother : ______________________
Education of the Husband : ______________________
Occupation of the Mother : ______________________
Occupation of the Husband : ______________________
Family Income Status : ______________________/month
Type of Family : ______________________
Socioeconomic Status : ______________________
Date of Last Antenatal Visit : ______________________
Name of the Doctor : ______________________
Name of the Primary Health Center : ______________________
Address : ______________________
____
____
____

Obstetrical Score : G ______ P ______ A ______ L ______ D ______ S ______
Age at Marriage : ______________________
Use of Contraceptives : ______________________
Relationship with Spouse : Consanguineous/Nonconsanguineous
Diagnosis, if any : ______________________

Family History

Type of family : ______________________
Congenital deformities : Present/Absent
Hereditary disease : Present/Absent

If present means mention : ____________________

____

____

Multiple pregnancies : ____________________

Menstrual History

Age at menarche : ____________________

Duration of menstrual cycles : ____________________

Menstrual cycle regularity : ____________________

Dysmenorrhea/Leukorrhea/
Menorrhagia : ____________________

____

Duration : ____________________

Last menstrual period : Date: __________ Month: __________

Present Obstetrical History

Period of gestational weeks : ____________________

Date of confirmation of pregnancy : ____________________

Last menstrual period : ____________________

Expected date of delivery : ____________________

Quickening : ____________________

Gravida : ____________________

Para : ____________________

Investigation

Sl No.	Investigation	Result

Minor disorders : ____________________

____

____

If any, specify : ____________________

____

____

Antenatal Examination

Parameters	1st month	2nd month	3rd month	4th month	5th month	6th month	7th month	8th month	9th month
Weight (kg)									
Weight increase (kg)									
Height (cm)									
Temperature									
Pulse									
Respiration									
Blood pressure									

Urine Test

Sugar : ____________________

Albumin : ____________________

Inspection

General appearance : ____________________

Stature (normal/short) : ____________________

Palpation

Fundal : ____________________

Abdominal girth : ____________________

Lateral : ____________________

Pelvic : ____________________

Auscultation

Fetal heart rate (FHR) : ____________________ Regular/Irregular

Past Obstetrical History

Year of last childbirth : ______________________

Number of children : ______________________

1	2	3	4

Type of delivery:
- Normal delivery (N)
- Cesarean section (CS)

1	2	3	4

Sex of the child:
- Male (M)
- Female (F)

1	2	3	4

Location : ______________________

Any complaints after delivery : ______________________

Sl No.	Age of the child	Type of delivery	Baby alive/dead	Sex of the baby	Birth weight of the baby	Any congenital deformities	Term	Abortion	Remarks
1.									
2.									
3.									
4.									
5.									

Physical Examination

Nourishment : ______________________

Body built : ______________________

Weight : ______________________kg

Height : ______________________cm

Vital signs

Temperature : ______________________

Pulse : ______________________

Respiration : ______________________

Blood pressure : ______________________

Mental status

Consciousness : ______________________

Look : ______________________

Head to Foot Examination

Skin turgor : ______________________

Moisture : ______________________

Warmth/Temperature : ______________________

Face : ______________________

Facial puffiness : ______________________

Lips : ______________________

Eyes : ______________________

Periorbital edema : ______________________

Conjunctiva : Pallor

Mouth : ______________________

Tongue : ______________________

Breast

Inspection : ______________________

____

____

Palpation : ______________________

____

____

Nipples : ______________________________
____
____

Abdomen:

Inspection

Size : ______________________________

Shape : ______________________________

Contour : ______________________________

Marks : ______________________________

Umbilicus : ______________________________

Fetal movements : ______________________________

Skin changes : ______________________________

Contractions : Present/Absent

Palpation

Fundal : Description

Inference : ______________________________

Lic : ______________________________

Presentation : ______________________________

Lateral

Left side : Description

Right side : Description inference: Position

Pelvic

First pelvic grip : ______________________________

Second pelvic grip : ______________________________

Inference

Position : ______________________________

Engagement/Not engagement : ______________________________

Attitude : ______________________________

Pawlik's grip : Fixed/Mobile

Auscultation

Fetal heart rate (FHR) : ______________________________

Rhythm : ______________________________

Location : ______________________________

Extremities

Ankle edema : __________

Capillary refill : __________

Cyanosis : __________

Palm fas delivery : __________

Health Education

Summary

Conclusion

Signature of the Student
Date:

Signature of the Clinical Coordinator
Date:

Antenatal Assessment

Case 5

Card Number ____________________

Mother Profile

Name of the Mother : ____________________
Age of the Mother : ____________________
Age of the Husband : ____________________
Education of the Mother : ____________________
Education of the Husband : ____________________
Occupation of the Mother : ____________________
Occupation of the Husband : ____________________
Family Income Status : ____________________/month
Type of Family : ____________________
Socioeconomic Status : ____________________
Date of Last Antenatal Visit : ____________________
Name of the Doctor : ____________________
Name of the Primary Health Center : ____________________
Address : ____________________
____
____
____

Obstetrical Score : G ______ P ______ A ______ L ______ D ______ S ______
Age at Marriage : ____________________
Use of Contraceptives : ____________________
Relationship with Spouse : Consanguineous/Nonconsanguineous
Diagnosis, if any : ____________________

Family History

Type of family : ____________________
Congenital deformities : Present/Absent
Hereditary disease : Present/Absent

If present means mention : ____________________

____

____

Multiple pregnancies : ____________________

Menstrual History

Age at menarche : ____________________

Duration of menstrual cycles : ____________________

Menstrual cycle regularity : ____________________

Dysmenorrhea/Leukorrhea/

Menorrhagia : ____________________

____

Duration : ____________________

Last menstrual period : Date: ____________ Month: ____________

Present Obstetrical History

Period of gestational weeks : ____________________

Date of confirmation of pregnancy : ____________________

Last menstrual period : ____________________

Expected date of delivery : ____________________

Quickening : ____________________

Gravida : ____________________

Para : ____________________

Investigation

Sl No.	Investigation	Result

Minor disorders : ____________________

____

____

If any, specify : ______________________

____

____

Antenatal Examination

Parameters	1st month	2nd month	3rd month	4th month	5th month	6th month	7th month	8th month	9th month
Weight (kg)									
Weight increase (kg)									
Height (cm)									
Temperature									
Pulse									
Respiration									
Blood pressure									

Urine Test

Sugar : ______________________

Albumin : ______________________

Inspection

General appearance : ______________________

Stature (normal/short) : ______________________

Palpation

Fundal : ______________________

Abdominal girth : ______________________

Lateral : ______________________

Pelvic : ______________________

Auscultation

Fetal heart rate (FHR) : ______________________ Regular/Irregular

Past Obstetrical History

Year of last childbirth : ______________________

Number of children : ______________________

1	2	3	4

Type of delivery:
- Normal delivery (N)
- Cesarean section (CS)

1	2	3	4

Sex of the child:
- Male (M)
- Female (F)

1	2	3	4

Location : ______________________

Any complaints after delivery : ______________________

Sl No.	Age of the child	Type of delivery	Baby alive/dead	Sex of the baby	Birth weight of the baby	Any congenital deformities	Term	Abortion	Remarks
1.									
2.									
3.									
4.									
5.									

Physical Examination

Nourishment : ____________________

Body built : ____________________

Weight : ____________________kg

Height : ____________________cm

Vital signs

Temperature : ____________________

Pulse : ____________________

Respiration : ____________________

Blood pressure : ____________________

Mental status

Consciousness : ____________________

Look : ____________________

Head to Foot Examination

Skin turgor : ____________________

Moisture : ____________________

Warmth/Temperature : ____________________

Face : ____________________

Facial puffiness : ____________________

Lips : ____________________

Eyes : ____________________

Periorbital edema : ____________________

Conjunctiva : Pallor

Mouth : ____________________

Tongue : ____________________

Breast

Inspection : ____________________

____

____

Palpation : ____________________

____

____

Nipples : ________________________________

____

____

Abdomen:

Inspection

Size : ________________________________

Shape : ________________________________

Contour : ________________________________

Marks : ________________________________

Umbilicus : ________________________________

Fetal movements : ________________________________

Skin changes : ________________________________

Contractions : Present/Absent

Palpation

Fundal : Description

Inference : ________________________________

Lic : ________________________________

Presentation : ________________________________

Lateral

Left side : Description

Right side : Description inference: Position

Pelvic

First pelvic grip : ________________________________

Second pelvic grip : ________________________________

Inference

Position : ________________________________

Engagement/Not engagement : ________________________________

Attitude : ________________________________

Pawlik's grip : Fixed/Mobile

Auscultation

Fetal heart rate (FHR) : ________________________________

Rhythm : ________________________________

Location : ________________________________

Extremities

Ankle edema : ________________________

Capillary refill : ________________________

Cyanosis : ________________________

Palm fas delivery : ________________________

Health Education

Summary

Conclusion

Signature of the Student
Date:

Signature of the Clinical Coordinator
Date:

Postnatal Assessment

Case 1

Identification Profile

Name of the Mother : __________
Age of the Mother : __________
Name of the Husband : __________
Age of the Husband : __________
Education of the Mother : __________
Education of the Husband : __________
Occupation of the Mother : __________
Occupation of the Husband : __________
Family Income Status : __________/month
Type of Family : __________
Socioeconomic Status : __________
Date and Time of Delivery : __________
Name of the Doctor/Dai to
Conduct Delivery : __________
Name of the Primary Health Center : __________
Address : __________

____

____

____

Age at Marriage : __________
Use of Contraceptives : __________
Relationship with Spouse : Consanguineous/Nonconsanguineous
Diagnosis, if any : __________

Personal and Family History

Dietary : __________
Habit : __________
Use of contraceptives : __________

Illness : Tuberculosis/Hypertension/Diabetics

Type of family : ____________________

Congenital deformities : Present/Absent

Hereditary disease : Present/Absent

If present means mention : ____________________

____

____

Multiple pregnancies : ____________________

Menstrual History

Age at menarche : ____________________

Duration of menstrual cycles : ____________________

Menstrual cycle regularity : ____________________

Dysmenorrhea/Leukorrhea/
Menorrhagia : ____________________

____

Duration : ____________________

Last menstrual period : Date: ____________ Month: ____________

Present Obstetrical History

Period of gestational weeks : ____________________

Date of confirmation of pregnancy : ____________________

Last menstrual period : ____________________

Expected date of delivery : ____________________

Quickening : ____________________

Gravida : ____________________

Para : ____________________

Blood group and Rh : ____________________

Investigation

Sl No.	Investigation	Result

Minor disorders : ______________________________

____

____

High-risk group : Yes/No (any specify)

____

____

Postnatal Examination

Parameters	1st week	2nd week	3rd week	4th week	5th week	6th week	7th week	8th week	9th week
Weight (kg)									
Height (cm)									
Temperature									
Pulse									
Respiration									
Blood pressure									

Urine Test

Sugar : ______________________________

Albumin : ______________________________

Date of delivery : ______________________________

Mode of delivery : ______________________________

Parity : ______________________________

Inspection

General appearance : ______________________________

Stature (normal/short) : ______________________________

Normal (vaginal) :

With episiotomy : ______________________________

Without episiotomy : ______________________________

Any tear : 1st degree/2nd degree/3rd degree

Spontaneous/Medical/

Cesarean/Any other : ______________________________

Full term/Preterm or Premature : ______________________________

Presentation : Vertex/Breech/Shoulder/Face: ____________________

Involution of uterus : ____________________

Palpation of delivery : ____________________

Past Obstetrical History

Type of delivery:

- Normal delivery (N)
- Cesarean section (CS)

1st	2nd	3rd	4th
Child	Child	Child	Child

Sex of the child:

- Male (M)
- Female (F)

1st	2nd	3rd	4th
Child	Child	Child	Child

Any complaints after delivery : ____________________

Sl No.	Age of the child	Type of delivery	Baby alive/dead	Sex of the baby	Birth weight of the baby	Any congenital deformities	Term	Abortion	Remarks
1.									
2.									
3.									
4.									
5.									

Physical Examination

Nourishment : Well-nourished/Undernourished
Body built : Thin/Obese
Weight : ____________kg
Height : ____________cm

Vital signs

Temperature : ____________°C
Pulse : ____________/minute
Respiration : ____________/minute
Blood pressure : ____________mm Hg

Mental status

Consciousness : Conscious/Unconscious/Delirious
Mood : Anxious/Worried/Depressed

Head to Foot Examination

Skin turgor : ____________
Moisture : ____________
Warmth/Temperature : ____________
Nails : ____________
Color : ____________
Capillary refill : ____________
Shapes : ____________

Face

Facial puffiness : ____________
Lips : ____________
Eyes : ____________
Conjunctiva : Pallor
Mouth : ____________
Tongue : ____________
Neck : ____________
Throat and pharynx : ____________
Thyroid gland : ____________

Chest

Thorax : ____________
Breath sound : ____________

Heart : __________

Axilla : __________

Breast : Secretion of colostrums/milk

Inspection : __________

Palpation : __________

Nipples : __________

Abdomen:

Inspection

Presence of scar/wound/if cesarean, discharge/tenderness presence of stria.

Palpation

Height of the uterus : __________cm

Consistency : Hard/Firm/Boggy

Auscultation

Bowel sound : __________

Perineum : Intact/Tear/Wound

Episiotomy : Mediolateral/Lateral/Medial

Condition of the wound : Redness/Edematous/Hematoma/Discharge/Approximation

Lochia : __________

Amount of bleeding : Scanty/Moderate/Heavy

Color : Red/Yellow/White/Rubra/Serosa/Alba__________

Odor : Fishy odor/Foul smelling

Clots : Present/Absent

Cervix : Edematous/Thin/Fragile

os : Open/Closed (any tear)

Vaginal mucosa : Smooth/Distended/Atrophic

Vaginal introitus : Erythematous/Edematous

Bladder function : __________

Hemorrhoids/Anal varicosities : Present/Absent

Ankle edema/Varicose vein : __________

Extremities : Generalized muscular fatigue

Homans' sign : Positive/Negative

Present History of Delivery

Mode of delivery : ______________________

Term of the baby : ______________________

Abortion : ______________________

Birth baby : Alive/Dead

Sex of the baby : ______________________

Birth weight : ______________________

Immunization

At birth : ______________________

Mother : ______________________

Initiation of breastfeeding : Yes/No

If no means specify : ______________________

Any abnormality : ______________________

Health Assessment of Newborn Baby

APGAR score : ______________________

Anthropometric measurement

Weight (kg) : ______________________

Length (cm) : ______________________

Head circumference : ______________________

Chest circumference : ______________________

Mid-arm circumference : ______________________

Anterior fontanel : ______________________

Posterior fontanel : ______________________

If any abnormality : ______________________

Health Education

____

____

____

____

Summary

Conclusion

Signature of the Student
Date:

Signature of the Clinical Coordinator
Date:

Signature of the HOD of Community Health Nursing
Date:

Postnatal Assessment

Case 2

Identification Profile

Name of the Mother : ______________________

Age of the Mother : ______________________

Name of the Husband : ______________________

Age of the Husband : ______________________

Education of the Mother : ______________________

Education of the Husband : ______________________

Occupation of the Mother : ______________________

Occupation of the Husband : ______________________

Family Income Status : ______________________/month

Type of Family : ______________________

Socioeconomic Status : ______________________

Date and Time of Delivery : ______________________

Name of the Doctor/Dai to Conduct Delivery : ______________________

Name of the Primary Health Center : ______________________

Address : ______________________

____

____

____

Age at Marriage : ______________________

Use of Contraceptives : ______________________

Relationship with Spouse : Consanguineous/Nonconsanguineous

Diagnosis, if any : ______________________

Personal and Family History

Dietary : ______________________

Habit : ______________________

Use of contraceptives : ______________________

Illness : Tuberculosis/Hypertension/Diabetics

Type of family : ______________________________

Congenital deformities : Present/Absent

Hereditary disease : Present/Absent

If present means mention : ______________________________

____

____

Multiple pregnancies : ______________________________

Menstrual History

Age at menarche : ______________________________

Duration of menstrual cycles : ______________________________

Menstrual cycle regularity : ______________________________

Dysmenorrhea/Leukorrhea/

Menorrhagia : ______________________________

____

Duration : ______________________________

Last menstrual period : Date: ______________ Month: ______________

Present Obstetrical History

Period of gestational weeks : ______________________________

Date of confirmation of pregnancy : ______________________________

Last menstrual period : ______________________________

Expected date of delivery : ______________________________

Quickening : ______________________________

Gravida : ______________________________

Para : ______________________________

Blood group and Rh : ______________________________

Investigation

Sl No.	Investigation	Result

Minor disorders : ______________________________

____

____

High-risk group : Yes/No (any specify)

____

____

Postnatal Examination

Parameters	1st week	2nd week	3rd week	4th week	5th week	6th week	7th week	8th week	9th week
Weight (kg)									
Height (cm)									
Temperature									
Pulse									
Respiration									
Blood pressure									

Urine Test

Sugar : ______________________________

Albumin : ______________________________

Date of delivery : ______________________________

Mode of delivery : ______________________________

Parity : ______________________________

Inspection

General appearance : ______________________________

Stature (normal/short) : ______________________________

Normal (vaginal) :

With episiotomy : ______________________________

Without episiotomy : ______________________________

Any tear : 1st degree/2nd degree/3rd degree

Spontaneous/Medical/

Cesarean/Any other : ______________________________

Full term/Preterm or Premature : ______________________________

Presentation : Vertex/Breech/Shoulder/Face: ____________________

Involution of uterus : ____________________

Palpation of delivery : ____________________

Past Obstetrical History

Type of delivery:
- Normal delivery (N)
- Cesarean section (CS)

1st	2nd	3rd	4th
Child	Child	Child	Child

Sex of the child:
- Male (M)
- Female (F)

1st	2nd	3rd	4th
Child	Child	Child	Child

Any complaints after delivery : ____________________

Sl No.	Age of the child	Type of delivery	Baby alive/dead	Sex of the baby	Birth weight of the baby	Any congenital deformities	Term	Abortion	Remarks
1.									
2.									
3.									
4.									
5.									

Physical Examination

Nourishment : Well-nourished/Undernourished

Body built : Thin/Obese

Weight : ____________________ kg

Height : ____________________ cm

Vital signs

Temperature : ____________________ °C

Pulse : ____________________ /minute

Respiration : ____________________ /minute

Blood pressure : ____________________ mm Hg

Mental status

Consciousness : Conscious/Unconscious/Delirious

Mood : Anxious/Worried/Depressed

Head to Foot Examination

Skin turgor : ____________________

Moisture : ____________________

Warmth/Temperature : ____________________

Nails : ____________________

Color : ____________________

Capillary refill : ____________________

Shapes : ____________________

Face

Facial puffiness : ____________________

Lips : ____________________

Eyes : ____________________

Conjunctiva : Pallor

Mouth : ____________________

Tongue : ____________________

Neck : ____________________

Throat and pharynx : ____________________

Thyroid gland : ____________________

Chest

Thorax : ____________________

Breath sound : ____________________

Heart : __________

Axilla : __________

Breast : Secretion of colostrums/milk

Inspection : __________

Palpation : __________

Nipples : __________

Abdomen:

Inspection

Presence of scar/wound/if cesarean, discharge/tenderness presence of stria.

Palpation

Height of the uterus : __________cm

Consistency : Hard/Firm/Boggy

Auscultation

Bowel sound : __________

Perineum : Intact/Tear/Wound

Episiotomy : Mediolateral/Lateral/Medial

Condition of the wound : Redness/Edematous/Hematoma/Discharge/Approximation

Lochia : __________

Amount of bleeding : Scanty/Moderate/Heavy

Color : Red/Yellow/White/Rubra/Serosa/Alba__________

Odor : Fishy odor/Foul smelling

Clots : Present/Absent

Cervix : Edematous/Thin/Fragile

os : Open/Closed (any tear)

Vaginal mucosa : Smooth/Distended/Atrophic

Vaginal introitus : Erythematous/Edematous

Bladder function : __________

Hemorrhoids/Anal varicosities : Present/Absent

Ankle edema/Varicose vein : __________

Extremities : Generalized muscular fatigue
Homans' sign : Positive/Negative

Present History of Delivery

Mode of delivery : ______________________________
Term of the baby : ______________________________
Abortion : ______________________________
Birth baby : Alive/Dead
Sex of the baby : ______________________________
Birth weight : ______________________________

Immunization

At birth : ______________________________
Mother : ______________________________
Initiation of breastfeeding : Yes/No
If no means specify : ______________________________
Any abnormality : ______________________________

Health Assessment of Newborn Baby

APGAR score : ______________________________
Anthropometric measurement
Weight (kg) : ______________________________
Length (cm) : ______________________________
Head circumference : ______________________________
Chest circumference : ______________________________
Mid-arm circumference : ______________________________
Anterior fontanel : ______________________________
Posterior fontanel : ______________________________
If any abnormality : ______________________________

Health Education

____

____

____

____

Summary

Conclusion

Signature of the Student
Date:

Signature of the Clinical Coordinator
Date:

Signature of the HOD of Community Health Nursing
Datc:

Postnatal Assessment

Case 3

Identification Profile

Name of the Mother : ____________________

Age of the Mother : ____________________

Name of the Husband : ____________________

Age of the Husband : ____________________

Education of the Mother : ____________________

Education of the Husband : ____________________

Occupation of the Mother : ____________________

Occupation of the Husband : ____________________

Family Income Status : ____________________/month

Type of Family : ____________________

Socioeconomic Status : ____________________

Date and Time of Delivery : ____________________

Name of the Doctor/Dai to Conduct Delivery : ____________________

Name of the Primary Health Center : ____________________

Address : ____________________

____

____

____

Age at Marriage : ____________________

Use of Contraceptives : ____________________

Relationship with Spouse : Consanguineous/Nonconsanguineous

Diagnosis, if any : ____________________

Personal and Family History

Dietary : ____________________

Habit : ____________________

Use of contraceptives : ____________________

Illness : Tuberculosis/Hypertension/Diabetics
Type of family : __________
Congenital deformities : Present/Absent
Hereditary disease : Present/Absent
If present means mention : __________

Multiple pregnancies : __________

Menstrual History

Age at menarche : __________
Duration of menstrual cycles : __________
Menstrual cycle regularity : __________
Dysmenorrhea/Leukorrhea/
Menorrhagia : __________

Duration : __________
Last menstrual period : Date: __________ Month: __________

Present Obstetrical History

Period of gestational weeks : __________
Date of confirmation of pregnancy : __________
Last menstrual period : __________
Expected date of delivery : __________
Quickening : __________
Gravida : __________
Para : __________
Blood group and Rh : __________

Investigation

Sl No.	Investigation	Result

Minor disorders : ______________________________

____

____

High-risk group : Yes/No (any specify)

____

____

Postnatal Examination

Parameters	1st week	2nd week	3rd week	4th week	5th week	6th week	7th week	8th week	9th week
Weight (kg)									
Height (cm)									
Temperature									
Pulse									
Respiration									
Blood pressure									

Urine Test

Sugar : ______________________________

Albumin : ______________________________

Date of delivery : ______________________________

Mode of delivery : ______________________________

Parity : ______________________________

Inspection

General appearance : ______________________________

Stature (normal/short) : ______________________________

Normal (vaginal) :

With episiotomy : ______________________________

Without episiotomy : ______________________________

Any tear : 1st degree/2nd degree/3rd degree

Spontaneous/Medical/

Cesarean/Any other : ______________________________

Full term/Preterm or Premature : ______________________________

Presentation : Vertex/Breech/Shoulder/Face: ____________________

Involution of uterus : ____________________

Palpation of delivery : ____________________

Past Obstetrical History

Type of delivery:

- Normal delivery (N)
- Cesarean section (CS)

1st	2nd	3rd	4th
Child	Child	Child	Child

Sex of the child:

- Male (M)
- Female (F)

1st	2nd	3rd	4th
Child	Child	Child	Child

Any complaints after delivery : ____________________

Sl No.	Age of the child	Type of delivery	Baby alive/dead	Sex of the baby	Birth weight of the baby	Any congenital deformities	Term	Abortion	Remarks
1.									
2.									
3.									
4.									
5.									

Physical Examination

Nourishment : Well-nourished/Undernourished

Body built : Thin/Obese

Weight : ________________________ kg

Height : ________________________ cm

Vital signs

Temperature : ________________________ °C

Pulse : ________________________ /minute

Respiration : ________________________ /minute

Blood pressure : ________________________ mm Hg

Mental status

Consciousness : Conscious/Unconscious/Delirious

Mood : Anxious/Worried/Depressed

Head to Foot Examination

Skin turgor : ________________________

Moisture : ________________________

Warmth/Temperature : ________________________

Nails : ________________________

Color : ________________________

Capillary refill : ________________________

Shapes : ________________________

Face

Facial puffiness : ________________________

Lips : ________________________

Eyes : ________________________

Conjunctiva : Pallor

Mouth : ________________________

Tongue : ________________________

Neck : ________________________

Throat and pharynx : ________________________

Thyroid gland : ________________________

Chest

Thorax : ________________________

Breath sound : ________________________

Heart : __________

Axilla : __________

Breast : Secretion of colostrums/milk

Inspection : __________

Palpation : __________

Nipples : __________

Abdomen:

Inspection

Presence of scar/wound/if cesarean, discharge/tenderness presence of stria.

Palpation

Height of the uterus : __________cm

Consistency : Hard/Firm/Boggy

Auscultation

Bowel sound : __________

Perineum : Intact/Tear/Wound

Episiotomy : Mediolateral/Lateral/Medial

Condition of the wound : Redness/Edematous/Hematoma/Discharge/Approximation

Lochia : __________

Amount of bleeding : Scanty/Moderate/Heavy

Color : Red/Yellow/White/Rubra/Serosa/Alba__________

Odor : Fishy odor/Foul smelling

Clots : Present/Absent

Cervix : Edematous/Thin/Fragile

os : Open/Closed (any tear)

Vaginal mucosa : Smooth/Distended/Atrophic

Vaginal introitus : Erythematous/Edematous

Bladder function : __________

Hemorrhoids/Anal varicosities : Present/Absent

Ankle edema/Varicose vein : __________

Extremities : Generalized muscular fatigue

Homans' sign : Positive/Negative

Present History of Delivery

Mode of delivery : ____________________

Term of the baby : ____________________

Abortion : ____________________

Birth baby : Alive/Dead

Sex of the baby : ____________________

Birth weight : ____________________

Immunization

At birth : ____________________

Mother : ____________________

Initiation of breastfeeding : Yes/No

If no means specify : ____________________

Any abnormality : ____________________

Health Assessment of Newborn Baby

APGAR score : ____________________

Anthropometric measurement

Weight (kg) : ____________________

Length (cm) : ____________________

Head circumference : ____________________

Chest circumference : ____________________

Mid-arm circumference : ____________________

Anterior fontanel : ____________________

Posterior fontanel : ____________________

If any abnormality : ____________________

Health Education

____

____

____

____

Summary

Conclusion

Signature of the Student
Date:

Signature of the Clinical Coordinator
Date:

Signature of the HOD of Community Health Nursing
Date:

Postnatal Assessment

Case 4

Identification Profile

Name of the Mother : ____________________

Age of the Mother : ____________________

Name of the Husband : ____________________

Age of the Husband : ____________________

Education of the Mother : ____________________

Education of the Husband : ____________________

Occupation of the Mother : ____________________

Occupation of the Husband : ____________________

Family Income Status : ____________________/month

Type of Family : ____________________

Socioeconomic Status : ____________________

Date and Time of Delivery : ____________________

Name of the Doctor/Dai to Conduct Delivery : ____________________

Name of the Primary Health Center : ____________________

Address : ____________________

____

____

____

Age at Marriage : ____________________

Use of Contraceptives : ____________________

Relationship with Spouse : Consanguineous/Nonconsanguineous

Diagnosis, if any : ____________________

Personal and Family History

Dietary : ____________________

Habit : ____________________

Use of contraceptives : ____________________

Illness : Tuberculosis/Hypertension/Diabetics
Type of family : ____________________
Congenital deformities : Present/Absent
Hereditary disease : Present/Absent
If present means mention : ____________________
____
____

Multiple pregnancies : ____________________

Menstrual History

Age at menarche : ____________________
Duration of menstrual cycles : ____________________
Menstrual cycle regularity : ____________________
Dysmenorrhea/Leukorrhea/
Menorrhagia : ____________________
____

Duration : ____________________
Last menstrual period : Date: ____________ Month: ____________

Present Obstetrical History

Period of gestational weeks : ____________________
Date of confirmation of pregnancy : ____________________
Last menstrual period : ____________________
Expected date of delivery : ____________________
Quickening : ____________________
Gravida : ____________________
Para : ____________________
Blood group and Rh : ____________________

Investigation

Sl No.	Investigation	Result

Minor disorders : ______________________________

____

____

High-risk group : Yes/No (any specify)

____

____

Postnatal Examination

Parameters	1st week	2nd week	3rd week	4th week	5th week	6th week	7th week	8th week	9th week
Weight (kg)									
Height (cm)									
Temperature									
Pulse									
Respiration									
Blood pressure									

Urine Test

Sugar : ______________________________

Albumin : ______________________________

Date of delivery : ______________________________

Mode of delivery : ______________________________

Parity : ______________________________

Inspection

General appearance : ______________________________

Stature (normal/short) : ______________________________

Normal (vaginal) :

With episiotomy : ______________________________

Without episiotomy : ______________________________

Any tear : 1st degree/2nd degree/3rd degree

Spontaneous/Medical/

Cesarean/Any other : ______________________________

Full term/Preterm or Premature : ______________________________

Presentation : Vertex/Breech/Shoulder/Face: ____________

Involution of uterus : ____________

Palpation of delivery : ____________

Past Obstetrical History

Type of delivery:

- Normal delivery (N)
- Cesarean section (CS)

1st	2nd	3rd	4th
Child	Child	Child	Child

Sex of the child:

- Male (M)
- Female (F)

1st	2nd	3rd	4th
Child	Child	Child	Child

Any complaints after delivery : ____________

Sl No.	Age of the child	Type of delivery	Baby alive/dead	Sex of the baby	Birth weight of the baby	Any congenital deformities	Term	Abortion	Remarks
1.									
2.									
3.									
4.									
5.									

Physical Examination

Nourishment : Well-nourished/Undernourished

Body built : Thin/Obese

Weight : ______________________ kg

Height : ______________________ cm

Vital signs

Temperature : ______________________ °C

Pulse : ______________________ /minute

Respiration : ______________________ /minute

Blood pressure : ______________________ mm Hg

Mental status

Consciousness : Conscious/Unconscious/Delirious

Mood : Anxious/Worried/Depressed

Head to Foot Examination

Skin turgor : ______________________

Moisture : ______________________

Warmth/Temperature : ______________________

Nails : ______________________

Color : ______________________

Capillary refill : ______________________

Shapes : ______________________

Face

Facial puffiness : ______________________

Lips : ______________________

Eyes : ______________________

Conjunctiva : Pallor

Mouth : ______________________

Tongue : ______________________

Neck : ______________________

Throat and pharynx : ______________________

Thyroid gland : ______________________

Chest

Thorax : ______________________

Breath sound : ______________________

Heart : ____________________

Axilla : ____________________

Breast : Secretion of colostrums/milk

Inspection : ____________________

Palpation : ____________________

Nipples : ____________________

Abdomen:

Inspection

Presence of scar/wound/if cesarean, discharge/tenderness presence of stria.

Palpation

Height of the uterus : ____________________cm

Consistency : Hard/Firm/Boggy

Auscultation

Bowel sound : ____________________

Perineum : Intact/Tear/Wound

Episiotomy : Mediolateral/Lateral/Medial

Condition of the wound : Redness/Edematous/Hematoma/Discharge/Approximation

Lochia : ____________________

Amount of bleeding : Scanty/Moderate/Heavy

Color : Red/Yellow/White/Rubra/Serosa/Alba____________________

Odor : Fishy odor/Foul smelling

Clots : Present/Absent

Cervix : Edematous/Thin/Fragile

os : Open/Closed (any tear)

Vaginal mucosa : Smooth/Distended/Atrophic

Vaginal introitus : Erythematous/Edematous

Bladder function : ____________________

Hemorrhoids/Anal varicosities : Present/Absent

Ankle edema/Varicose vein : ____________________

Extremities : Generalized muscular fatigue

Homans' sign : Positive/Negative

Present History of Delivery

Mode of delivery : ______________________

Term of the baby : ______________________

Abortion : ______________________

Birth baby : Alive/Dead

Sex of the baby : ______________________

Birth weight : ______________________

Immunization

At birth : ______________________

Mother : ______________________

Initiation of breastfeeding : Yes/No

If no means specify : ______________________

Any abnormality : ______________________

Health Assessment of Newborn Baby

APGAR score : ______________________

Anthropometric measurement

Weight (kg) : ______________________

Length (cm) : ______________________

Head circumference : ______________________

Chest circumference : ______________________

Mid-arm circumference : ______________________

Anterior fontanel : ______________________

Posterior fontanel : ______________________

If any abnormality : ______________________

Health Education

____

____

____

____

Summary

Conclusion

Signature of the Student
Date:

Signature of the Clinical Coordinator
Date:

Signature of the HOD of Community Health Nursing
Date:

Postnatal Assessment

Case 5

Identification Profile

Name of the Mother : ____________________

Age of the Mother : ____________________

Name of the Husband : ____________________

Age of the Husband : ____________________

Education of the Mother : ____________________

Education of the Husband : ____________________

Occupation of the Mother : ____________________

Occupation of the Husband : ____________________

Family Income Status : ____________________/month

Type of Family : ____________________

Socioeconomic Status : ____________________

Date and Time of Delivery : ____________________

Name of the Doctor/Dai to Conduct Delivery : ____________________

Name of the Primary Health Center : ____________________

Address : ____________________

____

____

____

Age at Marriage : ____________________

Use of Contraceptives : ____________________

Relationship with Spouse : Consanguineous/Nonconsanguineous

Diagnosis, if any : ____________________

Personal and Family History

Dietary : ____________________

Habit : ____________________

Use of contraceptives : ____________________

Illness : Tuberculosis/Hypertension/Diabetics

Type of family : ______________________

Congenital deformities : Present/Absent

Hereditary disease : Present/Absent

If present means mention : ______________________

____

____

Multiple pregnancies : ______________________

Menstrual History

Age at menarche : ______________________

Duration of menstrual cycles : ______________________

Menstrual cycle regularity : ______________________

Dysmenorrhea/Leukorrhea/

Menorrhagia : ______________________

____

Duration : ______________________

Last menstrual period : Date: ____________ Month: ____________

Present Obstetrical History

Period of gestational weeks : ______________________

Date of confirmation of pregnancy : ______________________

Last menstrual period : ______________________

Expected date of delivery : ______________________

Quickening : ______________________

Gravida : ______________________

Para : ______________________

Blood group and Rh : ______________________

Investigation

Sl No.	Investigation	Result

Minor disorders : ___________________________

____

____

High-risk group : Yes/No (any specify)

____

____

Postnatal Examination

Parameters	1st week	2nd week	3rd week	4th week	5th week	6th week	7th week	8th week	9th week
Weight (kg)									
Height (cm)									
Temperature									
Pulse									
Respiration									
Blood pressure									

Urine Test

Sugar : ___________________________

Albumin : ___________________________

Date of delivery : ___________________________

Mode of delivery : ___________________________

Parity : ___________________________

Inspection

General appearance : ___________________________

Stature (normal/short) : ___________________________

Normal (vaginal) :

With episiotomy : ___________________________

Without episiotomy : ___________________________

Any tear : 1st degree/2nd degree/3rd degree

Spontaneous/Medical/

Cesarean/Any other : ___________________________

Full term/Preterm or Premature : ___________________________

Presentation : Vertex/Breech/Shoulder/Face: ____________________

Involution of uterus : ____________________

Palpation of delivery : ____________________

Past Obstetrical History

Type of delivery:
- Normal delivery (N)
- Cesarean section (CS)

1st	2nd	3rd	4th
Child	Child	Child	Child

Sex of the child:
- Male (M)
- Female (F)

1st	2nd	3rd	4th
Child	Child	Child	Child

Any complaints after delivery : ____________________

Sl No.	Age of the child	Type of delivery	Baby alive/dead	Sex of the baby	Birth weight of the baby	Any congenital deformities	Term	Abortion	Remarks
1.									
2.									
3.									
4.									
5.									

Physical Examination

Nourishment : Well-nourished/Undernourished

Body built : Thin/Obese

Weight : ______________________ kg

Height : ______________________ cm

Vital signs

Temperature : ______________________ °C

Pulse : ______________________ /minute

Respiration : ______________________ /minute

Blood pressure : ______________________ mm Hg

Mental status

Consciousness : Conscious/Unconscious/Delirious

Mood : Anxious/Worried/Depressed

Head to Foot Examination

Skin turgor : ______________________

Moisture : ______________________

Warmth/Temperature : ______________________

Nails : ______________________

Color : ______________________

Capillary refill : ______________________

Shapes : ______________________

Face

Facial puffiness : ______________________

Lips : ______________________

Eyes : ______________________

Conjunctiva : Pallor

Mouth : ______________________

Tongue : ______________________

Neck : ______________________

Throat and pharynx : ______________________

Thyroid gland : ______________________

Chest

Thorax : ______________________

Breath sound : ______________________

Heart : __________

Axilla : __________

Breast : Secretion of colostrums/milk

Inspection : __________

Palpation : __________

Nipples : __________

Abdomen:

Inspection

Presence of scar/wound/if cesarean, discharge/tenderness presence of stria.

Palpation

Height of the uterus : __________ cm

Consistency : Hard/Firm/Boggy

Auscultation

Bowel sound : __________

Perineum : Intact/Tear/Wound

Episiotomy : Mediolateral/Lateral/Medial

Condition of the wound : Redness/Edematous/Hematoma/Discharge/Approximation

Lochia : __________

Amount of bleeding : Scanty/Moderate/Heavy

Color : Red/Yellow/White/Rubra/Serosa/Alba __________

Odor : Fishy odor/Foul smelling

Clots : Present/Absent

Cervix : Edematous/Thin/Fragile

os : Open/Closed (any tear)

Vaginal mucosa : Smooth/Distended/Atrophic

Vaginal introitus : Erythematous/Edematous

Bladder function : __________

Hemorrhoids/Anal varicosities : Present/Absent

Ankle edema/Varicose vein : __________

Extremities : Generalized muscular fatigue

Homans' sign : Positive/Negative

Present History of Delivery

Mode of delivery : ______

Term of the baby : ______

Abortion : ______

Birth baby : Alive/Dead

Sex of the baby : ______

Birth weight : ______

Immunization

At birth : ______

Mother : ______

Initiation of breastfeeding : Yes/No

If no means specify : ______

Any abnormality : ______

Health Assessment of Newborn Baby

APGAR score : ______

Anthropometric measurement

Weight (kg) : ______

Length (cm) : ______

Head circumference : ______

Chest circumference : ______

Mid-arm circumference : ______

Anterior fontanel : ______

Posterior fontanel : ______

If any abnormality : ______

Health Education

______

______

______

______

Summary

Conclusion

Signature of the Student
Date:

Signature of the Clinical Coordinator
Date:

Signature of the HOD of Community Health Nursing
Date:

Preschool Health Assessment

Case 1

Identification Data

Name of the Child : ______________________

Age : ______________________

Sex : ______________________

Date of Birth : ______________________

Mode of Delivery : ______________________

Place of Birth : ______________________

Date of Birth : ______________________

Condition of Birth : ______________________

Type of Birth : ______________________

Birth Weight : ______________________

Name of the Mother : ______________________

Name of the Father : ______________________

Educational Status

Father : ______________________

Mother : ______________________

Occupational Status

Father : ______________________

Mother : ______________________

Family income : ______________________

Address : ______________________

____

____

Growth and Development

Sl No.	Milestone	Actual development	Child's development
1.	Holds head erect	6th month	
2.	Sit with support	9th month	
3.	Crawling	9th month	
4.	Turns over	9th month	
5.	Stands with support	14th month	
6.	Walks with support	16th month	
7.	Walks without support	19th month	
8.	Runs	19th month	
9.	Brushes teeth	24th month	
10.	Washes self	24th month	
11.	Dresses self	30th month	
12.	Feeds self	36th month	
13.	Talks sentences	40th month	

Physical Examination

General appearance

Nourishment : ____________________

Body built : ____________________

Health : ____________________

Activity : ____________________

Mental status

Consciousness : ____________________

Look : ____________________

Vital signs

Temperature : ____________________°C

Pulse : ____________________/minute

Respiration : ____________________/minute

Blood pressure : ____________________mm Hg

Anthropometric measurement

Height/Length : ____________________

Weight : ____________________

Chest circumference : ____________________

Mid-arm circumference : ____________________

Body mass index (BMI) : ____________________

Skin condition : ____________________

Color : ____________________

Texture : ____________________

Temperature : ____________________

Lesion : ____________________

Sensation : ____________________

Head and face : ____________________

Scalp : ____________________

Face : ____________________

Hair color : ____________________

Eye : ____________________

Eyebrows : ____________________

Eyelashes : ____________________

Eyelids : ____________________

Eyeball : ____________________

Conjunctiva : ____________________

Lens : ____________________

Vision : ____________________

Nose : ____________________

External noses : ____________________

Nostrils : ____________________

Nasal septum : ____________________

Ear

External ear : ____________________

Tympanic membrane : ____________________

Hearing acuity : ____________________

Mouth

Lips : ____________________

Odor : ____________________

Teeth : ____________________

Tongue : ______________________

Speech : ______________________

Chest

Inspection : ______________________

Palpation : ______________________

Percussion : ______________________

Auscultation : ______________________

Abdomen

Inspection : ______________________

Palpation : ______________________

Auscultation : ______________________

Percussion : ______________________

Genitalia

: ______________________

____

Back : Mention any abnormal posturing: Lordosis/Scoliosis/Kyphosis

Impression : ______________________

Extremities : Present/Absent/Any illness (specify)

: ______________________

Immunization

Sl No.	Age	Vaccine	Given on	Remarks
1.				
2.				
3.				
4.				
5.				
6.				
7.				
8.				
9.				
10.				
11.				

Inference

Summary

Conclusion

Signature of the Student
Date:

Signature of the Clinical Instructor
Date:

Preschool Health Assessment

Case 2

Identification Data

Name of the Child : ____________________

Age : ____________________

Sex : ____________________

Date of Birth : ____________________

Mode of Delivery : ____________________

Place of Birth : ____________________

Date of Birth : ____________________

Condition of Birth : ____________________

Type of Birth : ____________________

Birth Weight : ____________________

Name of the Mother : ____________________

Name of the Father : ____________________

Educational Status

Father : ____________________

Mother : ____________________

Occupational Status

Father : ____________________

Mother : ____________________

Family income : ____________________

Address : ____________________

____

____

Growth and Development

Sl No.	Milestone	Actual development	Child's development
1.	Holds head erect	6th month	
2.	Sit with support	9th month	
3.	Crawling	9th month	
4.	Turns over	9th month	
5.	Stands with support	14th month	
6.	Walks with support	16th month	
7.	Walks without support	19th month	
8.	Runs	19th month	
9.	Brushes teeth	24th month	
10.	Washes self	24th month	
11.	Dresses self	30th month	
12.	Feeds self	36th month	
13.	Talks sentences	40th month	

Physical Examination

General appearance

Nourishment : ____________________

Body built : ____________________

Health : ____________________

Activity : ____________________

Mental status

Consciousness : ____________________

Look : ____________________

Vital signs

Temperature : ____________________°C

Pulse : ____________________/minute

Respiration : ____________________/minute

Blood pressure : ____________________mm Hg

Anthropometric measurement

Height/Length : ____________________

Weight : ____________________

Chest circumference : __________
Mid-arm circumference : __________
Body mass index (BMI) : __________
Skin condition : __________
Color : __________
Texture : __________
Temperature : __________
Lesion : __________
Sensation : __________
Head and face : __________
Scalp : __________
Face : __________
Hair color : __________
Eye : __________
Eyebrows : __________
Eyelashes : __________
Eyelids : __________
Eyeball : __________
Conjunctiva : __________
Lens : __________
Vision : __________
Nose : __________
External noses : __________
Nostrils : __________
Nasal septum : __________

Ear

External ear : __________
Tympanic membrane : __________
Hearing acuity : __________

Mouth

Lips : __________
Odor : __________
Teeth : __________

Tongue : ______

Speech : ______

Chest

Inspection : ______

Palpation : ______

Percussion : ______

Auscultation : ______

Abdomen

Inspection : ______

Palpation : ______

Auscultation : ______

Percussion : ______

Genitalia

: ______

______

Back : Mention any abnormal posturing: Lordosis/Scoliosis/Kyphosis

Impression : ______

Extremities : Present/Absent/Any illness (specify)

: ______

Immunization

Sl No.	Age	Vaccine	Given on	Remarks
1.				
2.				
3.				
4.				
5.				
6.				
7.				
8.				
9.				
10.				
11.				

Inference

Summary

Conclusion

Signature of the Student
Date:

Signature of the Clinical Instructor
Date:

Preschool Health Assessment

Case 3

Identification Data

Name of the Child : ____________________
Age : ____________________
Sex : ____________________
Date of Birth : ____________________
Mode of Delivery : ____________________
Place of Birth : ____________________
Date of Birth : ____________________
Condition of Birth : ____________________
Type of Birth : ____________________
Birth Weight : ____________________
Name of the Mother : ____________________
Name of the Father : ____________________

Educational Status

Father : ____________________
Mother : ____________________

Occupational Status

Father : ____________________
Mother : ____________________
Family income : ____________________
Address : ____________________
____
____

Growth and Development

Sl No.	Milestone	Actual development	Child's development
1.	Holds head erect	6th month	
2.	Sit with support	9th month	
3.	Crawling	9th month	
4.	Turns over	9th month	
5.	Stands with support	14th month	
6.	Walks with support	16th month	
7.	Walks without support	19th month	
8.	Runs	19th month	
9.	Brushes teeth	24th month	
10.	Washes self	24th month	
11.	Dresses self	30th month	
12.	Feeds self	36th month	
13.	Talks sentences	40th month	

Physical Examination

General appearance

Nourishment : ______________________

Body built : ______________________

Health : ______________________

Activity : ______________________

Mental status

Consciousness : ______________________

Look : ______________________

Vital signs

Temperature : ______________________°C

Pulse : ______________________/minute

Respiration : ______________________/minute

Blood pressure : ______________________mm Hg

Anthropometric measurement

Height/Length : ______________________

Weight : ______________________

Chest circumference : ______

Mid-arm circumference : ______

Body mass index (BMI) : ______

Skin condition : ______

Color : ______

Texture : ______

Temperature : ______

Lesion : ______

Sensation : ______

Head and face : ______

Scalp : ______

Face : ______

Hair color : ______

Eye : ______

Eyebrows : ______

Eyelashes : ______

Eyelids : ______

Eyeball : ______

Conjunctiva : ______

Lens : ______

Vision : ______

Nose : ______

External noses : ______

Nostrils : ______

Nasal septum : ______

Ear

External ear : ______

Tympanic membrane : ______

Hearing acuity : ______

Mouth

Lips : ______

Odor : ______

Teeth : ______

Tongue : ______

Speech : ______

Chest

Inspection : ______

Palpation : ______

Percussion : ______

Auscultation : ______

Abdomen

Inspection : ______

Palpation : ______

Auscultation : ______

Percussion : ______

Genitalia

: ______

______

Back : Mention any abnormal posturing: Lordosis/Scoliosis/Kyphosis

Impression : ______

Extremities : Present/Absent/Any illness (specify)

: ______

Immunization

Sl No.	Age	Vaccine	Given on	Remarks
1.				
2.				
3.				
4.				
5.				
6.				
7.				
8.				
9.				
10.				
11.				

Inference

Summary

Conclusion

Signature of the Student
Date:

Signature of the Clinical Instructor
Date:

Newborn Assessment

Case 1

Introduction

Identification Data

Name of the Baby :

Age :

Sex :

Date of Birth :

Name of the Mother :

Name of the Father :

Birth Weight :

Order of Birth :

Place of delivery :

Type of Delivery :

APGAR Score :

Sl No.	Parameters	Score
1.	Appearance (color)	
2.	Pulse rate (heart rate)	
3.	Grimace (reflex response to nasal catheter)	
4.	Activity	
5.	Respiration	

Anthropometric Measurement

Weight (kg) : ____________________

Height/Length (cm) : ____________________

Head circumference : ____________________

Chest circumference : ____________________

Mid-arm circumference : ____________________

Reflexes

Sl No.	Name of the reflexes	Remarks (absent/present)
1.	Rooting reflex	
2.	Sucking reflex	
3.	Gag reflex	
4.	Extrusion reflex	
5.	Yawning reflex	
6.	Palmar grasp reflex	
7.	Moro reflex	
8.	Startle reflex	
9.	Tonic neck reflex	
10.	Grasping reflex	
11.	Plantar reflex	
12.	Doll's eye reflex	
13.	Glabellar reflex	
14.	Corneal reflex	
15.	Swallowing reflex	
16.	Babinski reflex	
17.	Stepping reflex	
18.	Traction reflex	
19.	Perez reflex	

Newborn Assessment

Vital signs

Temperature : ____________________°C

Pulse : ____________________/minute

Respiration : ______________________________/minute

Blood pressure : ______________________________mm Hg

General appearance

Color of skin : ______________________________

Texture : ______________________________

Peripheral cyanosis : ______________________________

Lanugo : ______________________________

Anthropometric measurement

Height/Length : ______________________________

Weight : ______________________________

Head circumference : ______________________________

Chest circumference : ______________________________

Mid-arm circumference : ______________________________

Head and face

Size of head : ______________________________

Eyes

Eyebrows : ______________________________

Eyelids : ______________________________

Conjunctiva : ______________________________

Vision : ______________________________

Ear

Pinna : ______________________________

Tympanic membrane : ______________________________

Hearing activity : ______________________________

Mouth

Lips : ______________________________

Tongue : ______________________________

Cleft lip and cleft palate : ______________________________

Neck

Thyroid gland : ______________________________

Lymph nodes : ______________________________

Range of motion : ______________________________

Chest

Thorax : ____________________

Breath sound : ____________________

Heart sound : ____________________

Abdomen

Inspection : ____________________

Palpation : ____________________

Auscultation : ____________________

Extremities

Range of motion : ____________________

Absence of dislocation : ____________________

Back

If any deformities : ____________________

Genitalia

If any deformities : ____________________

Investigation

Sl No.	Investigation	Baby's value	Normal value	Remarks
1.				
2.				
3.				
4.				
5.				

Immunization

Sl No.	Age	Vaccine	Given on	Remarks
1.				
2.				
3.				
4.				
5.				
6.				

Contd...

Contd...

Sl No.	Age	Vaccine	Given on	Remarks
7.				
8.				
9.				
10.				

Summary

Conclusion

Signature of the Student
Date:

Signature of the Clinical Instructor
Date:

Newborn Assessment

Case 2

Introduction

Identification Data

Name of the Baby :

Age :

Sex :

Date of Birth :

Name of the Mother :

Name of the Father :

Birth Weight :

Order of Birth :

Place of delivery :

Type of Delivery :

APGAR Score :

Sl No.	Parameters	Score
1.	Appearance (color)	
2.	Pulse rate (heart rate)	
3.	Grimace (reflex response to nasal catheter)	
4.	Activity	
5.	Respiration	

Anthropometric Measurement

Weight (kg) : ____________________

Height/Length (cm) : ____________________

Head circumference : ____________________

Chest circumference : ____________________

Mid-arm circumference : ____________________

Reflexes

Sl No.	Name of the reflexes	Remarks (absent/present)
1.	Rooting reflex	
2.	Sucking reflex	
3.	Gag reflex	
4.	Extrusion reflex	
5.	Yawning reflex	
6.	Palmar grasp reflex	
7.	Moro reflex	
8.	Startle reflex	
9.	Tonic neck reflex	
10.	Grasping reflex	
11.	Plantar reflex	
12.	Doll's eye reflex	
13.	Glabellar reflex	
14.	Corneal reflex	
15.	Swallowing reflex	
16.	Babinski reflex	
17.	Stepping reflex	
18.	Traction reflex	
19.	Perez reflex	

Newborn Assessment

Vital signs

Temperature : ____________________°C

Pulse : ____________________/minute

Respiration : ________________________________/minute

Blood pressure : ________________________________mm Hg

General appearance

Color of skin : ________________________________

Texture : ________________________________

Peripheral cyanosis : ________________________________

Lanugo : ________________________________

Anthropometric measurement

Height/Length : ________________________________

Weight : ________________________________

Head circumference : ________________________________

Chest circumference : ________________________________

Mid-arm circumference : ________________________________

Head and face

Size of head : ________________________________

Eyes

Eyebrows : ________________________________

Eyelids : ________________________________

Conjunctiva : ________________________________

Vision : ________________________________

Ear

Pinna : ________________________________

Tympanic membrane : ________________________________

Hearing activity : ________________________________

Mouth

Lips : ________________________________

Tongue : ________________________________

Cleft lip and cleft palate : ________________________________

Neck

Thyroid gland : ________________________________

Lymph nodes : ________________________________

Range of motion : ________________________________

Chest

Thorax : ____________________

Breath sound : ____________________

Heart sound : ____________________

Abdomen

Inspection : ____________________

Palpation : ____________________

Auscultation : ____________________

Extremities

Range of motion : ____________________

Absence of dislocation : ____________________

Back

If any deformities : ____________________

Genitalia

If any deformities : ____________________

Investigation

Sl No.	Investigation	Baby's value	Normal value	Remarks
1.				
2.				
3.				
4.				
5.				

Immunization

Sl No.	Age	Vaccine	Given on	Remarks
1.				
2.				
3.				
4.				
5.				
6.				

Contd...

Contd...

Sl No.	Age	Vaccine	Given on	Remarks
7.				
8.				
9.				
10.				

Summary

Conclusion

Signature of the Student
Date:

Signature of the Clinical Instructor
Date:

Newborn Assessment

Case 3

Introduction

____

____

____

____

____

____

____

____

Identification Data

Name of the Baby : ______________________

Age : ______________________

Sex : ______________________

Date of Birth : ______________________

Name of the Mother : ______________________

Name of the Father : ______________________

Birth Weight : ______________________

Order of Birth : ______________________

Place of delivery : ______________________

Type of Delivery : ______________________

APGAR Score : ______________________

Sl No.	Parameters	Score
1.	Appearance (color)	
2.	Pulse rate (heart rate)	
3.	Grimace (reflex response to nasal catheter)	
4.	Activity	
5.	Respiration	

Anthropometric Measurement

Weight (kg) : ____________________

Height/Length (cm) : ____________________

Head circumference : ____________________

Chest circumference : ____________________

Mid-arm circumference : ____________________

Reflexes

Sl No.	Name of the reflexes	Remarks (absent/present)
1.	Rooting reflex	
2.	Sucking reflex	
3.	Gag reflex	
4.	Extrusion reflex	
5.	Yawning reflex	
6.	Palmar grasp reflex	
7.	Moro reflex	
8.	Startle reflex	
9.	Tonic neck reflex	
10.	Grasping reflex	
11.	Plantar reflex	
12.	Doll's eye reflex	
13.	Glabellar reflex	
14.	Corneal reflex	
15.	Swallowing reflex	
16.	Babinski reflex	
17.	Stepping reflex	
18.	Traction reflex	
19.	Perez reflex	

Newborn Assessment

Vital signs

Temperature : ____________________°C

Pulse : ____________________/minute

Respiration : ______________________________/minute

Blood pressure : ______________________________mm Hg

General appearance

Color of skin : ______________________________

Texture : ______________________________

Peripheral cyanosis : ______________________________

Lanugo : ______________________________

Anthropometric measurement

Height/Length : ______________________________

Weight : ______________________________

Head circumference : ______________________________

Chest circumference : ______________________________

Mid-arm circumference : ______________________________

Head and face

Size of head : ______________________________

Eyes

Eyebrows : ______________________________

Eyelids : ______________________________

Conjunctiva : ______________________________

Vision : ______________________________

Ear

Pinna : ______________________________

Tympanic membrane : ______________________________

Hearing activity : ______________________________

Mouth

Lips : ______________________________

Tongue : ______________________________

Cleft lip and cleft palate : ______________________________

Neck

Thyroid gland : ______________________________

Lymph nodes : ______________________________

Range of motion : ______________________________

Chest

Thorax : ____________________

Breath sound : ____________________

Heart sound : ____________________

Abdomen

Inspection : ____________________

Palpation : ____________________

Auscultation : ____________________

Extremities

Range of motion : ____________________

Absence of dislocation : ____________________

Back

If any deformities : ____________________

Genitalia

If any deformities : ____________________

Investigation

Sl No.	Investigation	Baby's value	Normal value	Remarks
1.				
2.				
3.				
4.				
5.				

Immunization

Sl No.	Age	Vaccine	Given on	Remarks
1.				
2.				
3.				
4.				
5.				
6.				

Contd...

Contd...

Sl No.	Age	Vaccine	Given on	Remarks
7.				
8.				
9.				
10.				

Summary

Conclusion

Signature of the Student
Date:

Signature of the Clinical Instructor
Date:

Old Age Assessment

Case 1

Personal Data

Name of the Person : ____________________

Age : ____________________

Sex : ____________________

Marital Status : ____________________

Type of Family : ____________________

Educational Status : ____________________

Occupational Status : ____________________

Income of the Family : ____________________

Nature of the House : ____________________

Permanent Address : ____________________

Personal History

Dietary habit : ____________________

Habits of daily activities : ____________________

Daily healthy practice : ____________________

Hobbies : ____________________

Name of the caretaker : ____________________

Relationship of the person : ____________________

Number of sons/daughters : ____________________

Name of the family doctor : ____________________

Phone number of the doctor : ____________________

Place of taking treatment : ____________________

Present complaint of person : ____________________

Health History

Present Medical History

History of Adult Illness

Past Medical History

Frequency of Doctors Visits

Physical Examination

General Appearance

Head to Foot Assessment

Face and neck

Unhealed sore, mole
or irregularly shaped lesion : ______

Skin : Dry/Oily/Normal ______

Loosen skin : Present/Absent

Finger nail : Soft/Thickened

Eyes

Color : ______

Tearing : Present/Absent

Vision : Night vision/Double vision/Blurred vision/
Corrective lenses/Glaucoma/Cataract

Ear

Ear pain : ______

Tinnitus : ______

Ear discharge : ______

Hearing problems : ______

Nose

Deviation : ______

Running : ______

Blocked : ______

Tongue : ______

Throat

Color of throat : ______

Any signs and symptoms of infection : ______

Neck

Lymph node enlargement : ______

Any white patches on cheek : ______

Neck veins distention : ______

Respiratory system

Shape of the chest : Barrel/Pigeon/Cylindrical

Auscultation

Lung or breath problems : Present/Absent

Shortness of breath : Present/Absent

Excessive cough : Yes/No

Hemoptysis : Present/Absent

Breath sounds : ______________________

Heart sounds : ______________________

Percussion

Fluid collection : Present/Absent

Air collection : Present/Absent

Any special signs and symptoms present in the system : ______________________

____

____

Cardiovascular system

Weight : ______________________

Chest pain : ______________________

Activities of daily living (ADL) : ______________________

Frequent cough : Present/Absent

Wheezing/Dyspnea : Present/Absent

Gastrointestinal system

Sense of taste : ______________________

Wears dentures : ______________________

Difficulty in swallowing : ______________________

Rectal bleeding : ______________________

Any devices (feeding tube, parenteral nutrition or ostomy) : ______________________

____

____

Genitourinary system

Incontinence of urine : Present/Absent

Urinary infection : Present/Absent

Prostatic obstruction : Present/Absent

Decrease in the size of force of urine stream : ______________________

Dribbling after urination : Present/Absent

Female patient

Vaginal itching/discharge with pain : Present/Absent

Monthly breast self-examination : Done/Not done

Postmenopausal bleeding : Present/Absent

Neurological system

Coordination : ____________________

Strength or sensory perception : ____________________

Headache or seizures : ____________________

Syncope (loss of consciousness) : ____________________

Dizziness : ____________________

Memory loss or forgetfulness : ____________________

Musculoskeletal system

Fall : ____________________

Wearing prosthesis : ____________________

Joint pain : ____________________

Lower back pain : ____________________

Osteoarthritis : ____________________

Hematological and immune system

Joint pain/Weakness or fatigue : Present/Absent

Determine daily diet : ____________________

____

____

Current medication : ____________________

____

____

Adverse effect of medication : ____________________

____

____

Psychosocial assessment

Alcohol and tobacco : ____________________

Difficulty sleeping : ____________________

Sadness or depression : ____________________

Loss of interest in usual activities : ____________________

Mood : ____________________

Employment status : ______________________

Hobbies : ______________________

Sexual activities : ______________________

ADL assessment

Eating habits : ______________________

Sleeping pattern : ______________________

Mobility : ______________________

Food, cloth and shelter : ______________________

Finding of Abnormalities

Health Education

Summary

Conclusion

Signature of the Student
Date:

Signature of the Clinical Instructor
Date:

Old Age Assessment

Case 2

Personal Data

Name of the Person : ______

Age : ______

Sex : ______

Marital Status : ______

Type of Family : ______

Educational Status : ______

Occupational Status : ______

Income of the Family : ______

Nature of the House : ______

Permanent Address : ______

______

______

______

Personal History

Dietary habit : ______

Habits of daily activities : ______

Daily healthy practice : ______

Hobbies : ______

Name of the caretaker : ______

Relationship of the person : ______

Number of sons/daughters : ______

Name of the family doctor : ______

Phone number of the doctor : ______

Place of taking treatment : ______

Present complaint of person : ______

______

______

Health History

Present Medical History

History of Adult Illness

Past Medical History

Frequency of Doctors Visits

Physical Examination

General Appearance

Head to Foot Assessment

Face and neck

Unhealed sore, mole or irregularly shaped lesion	: ________________
Skin	: Dry/Oily/Normal ________________
Loosen skin	: Present/Absent
Finger nail	: Soft/Thickened

Eyes

Color	: ________________
Tearing	: Present/Absent
Vision	: Night vision/Double vision/Blurred vision/ Corrective lenses/Glaucoma/Cataract

Ear

Ear pain	: ________________
Tinnitus	: ________________
Ear discharge	: ________________
Hearing problems	: ________________

Nose

Deviation	: ________________
Running	: ________________
Blocked	: ________________
Tongue	: ________________

Throat

Color of throat	: ________________
Any signs and symptoms of infection	: ________________

Neck

Lymph node enlargement	: ________________
Any white patches on cheek	: ________________
Neck veins distention	: ________________

Respiratory system

Shape of the chest	: Barrel/Pigeon/Cylindrical

Auscultation

Lung or breath problems	: Present/Absent
Shortness of breath	: Present/Absent

Excessive cough : Yes/No

Hemoptysis : Present/Absent

Breath sounds : ____________________

Heart sounds : ____________________

Percussion

Fluid collection : Present/Absent

Air collection : Present/Absent

Any special signs and symptoms present in the system : ____________________

____

____

Cardiovascular system

Weight : ____________________

Chest pain : ____________________

Activities of daily living (ADL) : ____________________

Frequent cough : Present/Absent

Wheezing/Dyspnea : Present/Absent

Gastrointestinal system

Sense of taste : ____________________

Wears dentures : ____________________

Difficulty in swallowing : ____________________

Rectal bleeding : ____________________

Any devices (feeding tube, parenteral nutrition or ostomy) : ____________________

____

____

Genitourinary system

Incontinence of urine : Present/Absent

Urinary infection : Present/Absent

Prostatic obstruction : Present/Absent

Decrease in the size of force of urine stream : ____________________

Dribbling after urination : Present/Absent

Female patient

Vaginal itching/discharge with pain : Present/Absent

Monthly breast self-examination : Done/Not done

Postmenopausal bleeding : Present/Absent

Neurological system

Coordination : ______

Strength or sensory perception : ______

Headache or seizures : ______

Syncope (loss of consciousness) : ______

Dizziness : ______

Memory loss or forgetfulness : ______

Musculoskeletal system

Fall : ______

Wearing prosthesis : ______

Joint pain : ______

Lower back pain : ______

Osteoarthritis : ______

Hematological and immune system

Joint pain/Weakness or fatigue : Present/Absent

Determine daily diet : ______

______

______

Current medication : ______

______

______

Adverse effect of medication : ______

______

______

Psychosocial assessment

Alcohol and tobacco : ______

Difficulty sleeping : ______

Sadness or depression : ______

Loss of interest in usual activities : ______

Mood : ______

Employment status : ______

Hobbies : ______

Sexual activities : ______

ADL assessment

Eating habits : ______

Sleeping pattern : ______

Mobility : ______

Food, cloth and shelter : ______

Finding of Abnormalities

Health Education

Summary

Conclusion

Signature of the Student
Date:

Signature of the Clinical Instructor
Date:

Old Age Assessment

Case 3

Personal Data

Name of the Person : ______________________

Age : ______________________

Sex : ______________________

Marital Status : ______________________

Type of Family : ______________________

Educational Status : ______________________

Occupational Status : ______________________

Income of the Family : ______________________

Nature of the House : ______________________

Permanent Address : ______________________

____

____

____

Personal History

Dietary habit : ______________________

Habits of daily activities : ______________________

Daily healthy practice : ______________________

Hobbies : ______________________

Name of the caretaker : ______________________

Relationship of the person : ______________________

Number of sons/daughters : ______________________

Name of the family doctor : ______________________

Phone number of the doctor : ______________________

Place of taking treatment : ______________________

Present complaint of person : ______________________

____

____

Health History

Present Medical History

History of Adult Illness

Past Medical History

Frequency of Doctors Visits

Physical Examination

General Appearance

Head to Foot Assessment

Face and neck

Unhealed sore, mole or irregularly shaped lesion : ______________________________

Skin : Dry/Oily/Normal ______________________________

Loosen skin : Present/Absent

Finger nail : Soft/Thickened

Eyes

Color : ______________________________

Tearing : Present/Absent

Vision : Night vision/Double vision/Blurred vision/ Corrective lenses/Glaucoma/Cataract

Ear

Ear pain : ______________________________

Tinnitus : ______________________________

Ear discharge : ______________________________

Hearing problems : ______________________________

Nose

Deviation : ______________________________

Running : ______________________________

Blocked : ______________________________

Tongue : ______________________________

Throat

Color of throat : ______________________________

Any signs and symptoms of infection : ______________________________

Neck

Lymph node enlargement : ______________________________

Any white patches on cheek : ______________________________

Neck veins distention : ______________________________

Respiratory system

Shape of the chest : Barrel/Pigeon/Cylindrical

Auscultation

Lung or breath problems : Present/Absent

Shortness of breath : Present/Absent

Excessive cough : Yes/No
Hemoptysis : Present/Absent
Breath sounds : ______
Heart sounds : ______

Percussion

Fluid collection : Present/Absent
Air collection : Present/Absent
Any special signs and symptoms present in the system : ______

Cardiovascular system

Weight : ______
Chest pain : ______
Activities of daily living (ADL) : ______
Frequent cough : Present/Absent
Wheezing/Dyspnea : Present/Absent

Gastrointestinal system

Sense of taste : ______
Wears dentures : ______
Difficulty in swallowing : ______
Rectal bleeding : ______
Any devices (feeding tube, parenteral nutrition or ostomy) : ______

Genitourinary system

Incontinence of urine : Present/Absent
Urinary infection : Present/Absent
Prostatic obstruction : Present/Absent
Decrease in the size of force of urine stream : ______
Dribbling after urination : Present/Absent

Female patient

Vaginal itching/discharge with pain : Present/Absent

Monthly breast self-examination : Done/Not done

Postmenopausal bleeding : Present/Absent

Neurological system

Coordination : ____________________

Strength or sensory perception : ____________________

Headache or seizures : ____________________

Syncope (loss of consciousness) : ____________________

Dizziness : ____________________

Memory loss or forgetfulness : ____________________

Musculoskeletal system

Fall : ____________________

Wearing prosthesis : ____________________

Joint pain : ____________________

Lower back pain : ____________________

Osteoarthritis : ____________________

Hematological and immune system

Joint pain/Weakness or fatigue : Present/Absent

Determine daily diet : ____________________

____

____

Current medication : ____________________

____

____

Adverse effect of medication : ____________________

____

____

Psychosocial assessment

Alcohol and tobacco : ____________________

Difficulty sleeping : ____________________

Sadness or depression : ____________________

Loss of interest in usual activities : ____________________

Mood : ____________________

Employment status : ______________________
Hobbies : ______________________
Sexual activities : ______________________

ADL assessment

Eating habits : ______________________
Sleeping pattern : ______________________
Mobility : ______________________
Food, cloth and shelter : ______________________

Finding of Abnormalities

Health Education

Summary

Conclusion

Signature of the Student
Date:

Signature of the Clinical Instructor
Date:

Nutritional Assessment of Under-five Children

Case 1

Name of the Village/Area : ____________________

House Number : ____________________

Name of the Family Head : ____________________

Age/Sex : ____________________

Educational Status : ____________________

Occupational Status : ____________________

Address : ____________________

____

____

Common Cooking Method : Steaming/Boiling/Deep/Shallow frying

Preparation of Food : Hygienic/Unhygienic

Commonly Consuming Food Items : ____________________

____

Particulars of Parents

Sl No.	Name of the parents	Age	Sex	Education	Occupation	Remarks
1.						
2.						

Number of living children : ____________________

Sl No.	Name of the children	Order of live birth	Date of birth	Age	Sex	Education
1.						
2.						
3.						

Anthropometric Measurement

Weight (kg) : ____________________

Height/Length (cm) : ____________________

Head circumference (cm) : ____________________

Chest circumference (cm) : ______________________

Mid-arm circumference (cm) : ______________________

Degree of Malnutrition

____

____

____

____

____

____

Body Mass Index

____

____

____

____

____

____

Growth Chart

24-hour Dietary Recall Survey

Name of the area : ______

Taluk : ______

District : ______

Religion : ______

Total number of family members : ______

Family income : ______

Family Characteristics

Sl No.	Name	Age	Occupation			Vegetarian	Nonvegetarian
			Sedentary	Moderate	Hard		
1.							
2.							
3.							
4.							
5.							
6.							

Purchase of Raw Material and their Expenditure Per Day

Items	How often purchasing?			Monthly	Seasonally	Quantity	Expenditure per day
	Daily	By weekly	Weekly				
Cereals							
Pulses							
Milk							
Fruits							
Vegetables							
Jaggery							
Sugar							
Ghee							
Oil							
Eggs							
Meat							
Fish							

Shopping facilities : Markets/Village shop/Stores/Any other forms

Preservation of raw foods : Store room/Kitchen/No store/Living room

Preservation of cooked food : Refrigerator/Cupboard/Kitchen

Fuel used for cooking : Cooking gas/Electrical stove/Firewood/Kerosene stove

Do you have:

Vegetable garden? ____________________

Fruit tree? ____________________

Household Animals

Cow : ____________________

Buffalo : ____________________

Hen : ____________________

Goat : ____________________

Pig : ____________________

Nutrition Cycle of the Family

Items/Days	Items in gram							Average daily intake	Category
	1	2	3	4	5	6	7		
Wheat									Cereals
Rice									
Jowar									
Bajara									
Other									
Toor dal									Pulses
Arhar									
Urad									
Moong									
Green gram									
Ground nuts									
Others									
Milk									Milk products
Curd									

Contd...

Contd...

Items/Days	Items in gram							Average daily intake	Category
	1	2	3	4	5	6	7		
Buttermilk									
Others									
Oil									Fats
Ghee									
Dalda									
Leafy vegetables									Vegetables
Root/Tubers									
Others									
Tea									Beverage
Coffee									
Others									
Sugar									Sweeteners
Jaggery									
Meat									Animals foods
Fish									
Egg									
Banana									Fruits
Orange									
Papaya									
Pineapple									
Grapes									
Apple									
Guava									
Others									

Inference

____

____

____

WHO recommended nutritive values for commonly used food items in India

Sl No.	Food preparation	Quantity per serving	Weight per serving	Calories (kcal)	Protein (g)	Fat (g)	Carbohydrates (g)	Calcium (g)	Phosphorus (g)	Iron (mg)
Cereal and millet preparation										
I	*Rice preparation*									
1.	Plain rice	2 serving	504	595	11.9	0.9	134.8	0.02	0.2	11.9
2.	Sambar rice	1 serving	485	405	13.5	13.5	76.2	0.08	0.16	13.5
3.	Curd rice	1 serving	253	221	6	7	33.3	0.57	0.10	6
4.	Sweet rice	1 serving	177	432	3.6	12	77.4	0.01	0.05	3.6
5.	Idli	2 pcs	136	130	4.6	0.2	27.6	0.03	0.08	4.6
6.	Plain dosa	2 pcs	100	216	4.1	9.7	28.2	0.03	0.07	4 1
7.	Masala dosa	2 pcs	100	212	4.6	8 4	29.4	0.04	0.08	4.6
8.	Pongal (hot)	1 serving	148	200	5.5	6	30.5	0.03	0.07	5.5
9.	Adai (hot)	1 pc	96	195	6.6	4.4	31.8	0.03	0.09	6.6
II	*Wheat preparation*									
1.	Wheat upma	1 serving	128	163	3.8	5.4	24.7	0.01	0.04	0.7
2.	Chapatis	2 pcs	57	196	5	5.5	30.8	0.13	0.02	3
3.	Puris	2 pcs	32	136	2.2	8.4	13	0.06	0.01	1.3
4.	Plain parathas	1 pc	66	104	4.5	19.6	27.3	0.12	0.01	2.7
5.	Rava (dosa, idli)	2 pcs	114	212	5	8.5	28.7	0	0.06	0.9
6.	Kesari bath	1 serving	90	284	2	14.6	35.3	0.02	0.04	0.44
7.	Luchi	2 pcs	71	346	4	24	28	0.03	0.01	0.4
III	*Millet preparation*									
1.	Ragi balls	1 pc	336	446	6	7.6	86.8	0.3	0.4	6
2.	Ragi roti	2 pcs	185	460	8	9	87	0.3	0.4	6
3.	Maize roti	2 pcs	142	314	9.6	5.5	56.4	0.3	0.1	1.8
4.	Jowar roti	2 pcs	150	252	7.5	1.3	52.5	0.2	0.02	4.5
5.	Ragi puttu	1 serving	146	422	4.4	7.4	84	0.2	0.02	
IV	*Pulse preparation*									
1.	Bengal gram dal (cooked)	1½ cup	157	284	9	16.4	25.2	0.07	0.13	3.8
2.	Bengal gram dal	1 cup	154	178	3.2	35.9	44.7	0.09	0.08	0.4

Contd...

Contd...

Sl No.	Food preparation	Quantity per serving	Weight per serving	Calories (kcal)	Protein (g)	Fat (g)	Carbohydrates (g)	Calcium (g)	Phosphorus (g)	Iron (mg)
3.	Green gram dal (cooked)	1½ cup	142	171	7	7.7	18.4	0.08	0.09	2.7
4.	Red gram dal (cooked)	1½ cup	96	110	6.4	2	16.4	0.05	0.07	2.6
5.	Dal rasam	1½ cup	196	29	1.5	0.9	3.8	0.03	0.03	0.09
6.	Radish sambar (sundal)		196	101	4.1	3.6	13.1	0.04	0.07	2.2
7.	Green gram sambar (sundal)	1 cup	142	255	13.5	8.8	30.3	0.05	0.2	2.5
8.	Cowpea sundal	1 cup	142	259	13.1	9.2	30.9	0.08	0.2	4.8
9.	Amaranth sambar	1½ cup	140	250	5.1	2.7	13	0.05	0.08	8
10.	Bengal gram (sundal)	1 cup	142	272	13.2	11.1	29.7	0.11	0.15	5.5
V	*Vegetable preparation*									
1.	Amaranth curry	1½ plate	28	47	1.4	2.3	5.1	0.04	0.04	6.64
2.	Amaranth masala	½ plate	42	46	1.2	2.6	4.4	0.05	0.05	6.8
3.	Brinjal curry	½ plate	45	122	1.4	10.7	4.9	0.02	0.05	0.9
4.	Milk (buffalo)	1 cup	200	216	8.4	16	9.2	0.42	0.030	0.8
5.	Cabbage and carrot curry	½ plate	56	81	1.5	5.6	6.1	0.04	0.12	0.9
6.	Buttermilk	1 cup	200	36	1.8	2.8	2	0.07	0.07	0.2
7.	Buttermilk (buffalo)	1 cup	200	66	24	5.4	2.8	0.07	0.07	0.2
VI	*Egg, milk and meat preparation*									
1.	Meat curry	1 serving	128	220	116	18	2.7	0.1	0.01	2.1
2.	Omelet	1 serving	39	77	5.8	5.7	0.5	0.03	0.1	1
3.	Meat fry	1 serving	142	339	21.8	26	4.5	0.23	0.2	3.3
4.	Fish fry	1 serving	100	220	16.2	16.2	1.4	0.05	0.45	1.2
5.	Rice, mutton pulao	2 servings	341	686	39	39	63.6	0.1	0.22	1.5
VII	*Preparation containing milk*									
1.	Coffee	1 cup	200	104	3.8	3.4	14.4	0.1	0.1	1.2
2.	Tea	1 cup	200	72	1.4	1.6	13	0.06	0.04	-
3.	Cocoa	1 cup	200	174	7.5	20.2	20.2	0.2	0.15	0.3
4.	Wheat payasam	1 cup	154	178	3.4	31.5	31.5	0.09	0.08	0.4
5.	Rice payasam	1 cup	266	227	3.7	44.3	44.3	0.14	0.1	4.7
6.	Rice porridge	1 cup	280	263	7.6	44.7	35.9	0.3	0.2	0.7
7.	Soy porridge	1 cup	154	178	7.7	44	44.7	0.07	0.14	0.4
8.	Wheat porridge	1 cup	280	263	7.6	44.7	35.9	0.3	0.22	0.7
9.	Ragi porridge	1 cup	193	317	8.7	52.7	35.9	0.24	0.22	1
10.	Milk (cow)	1 cup	200	130	7	9.8	52.7	0.12	0.1	0.4

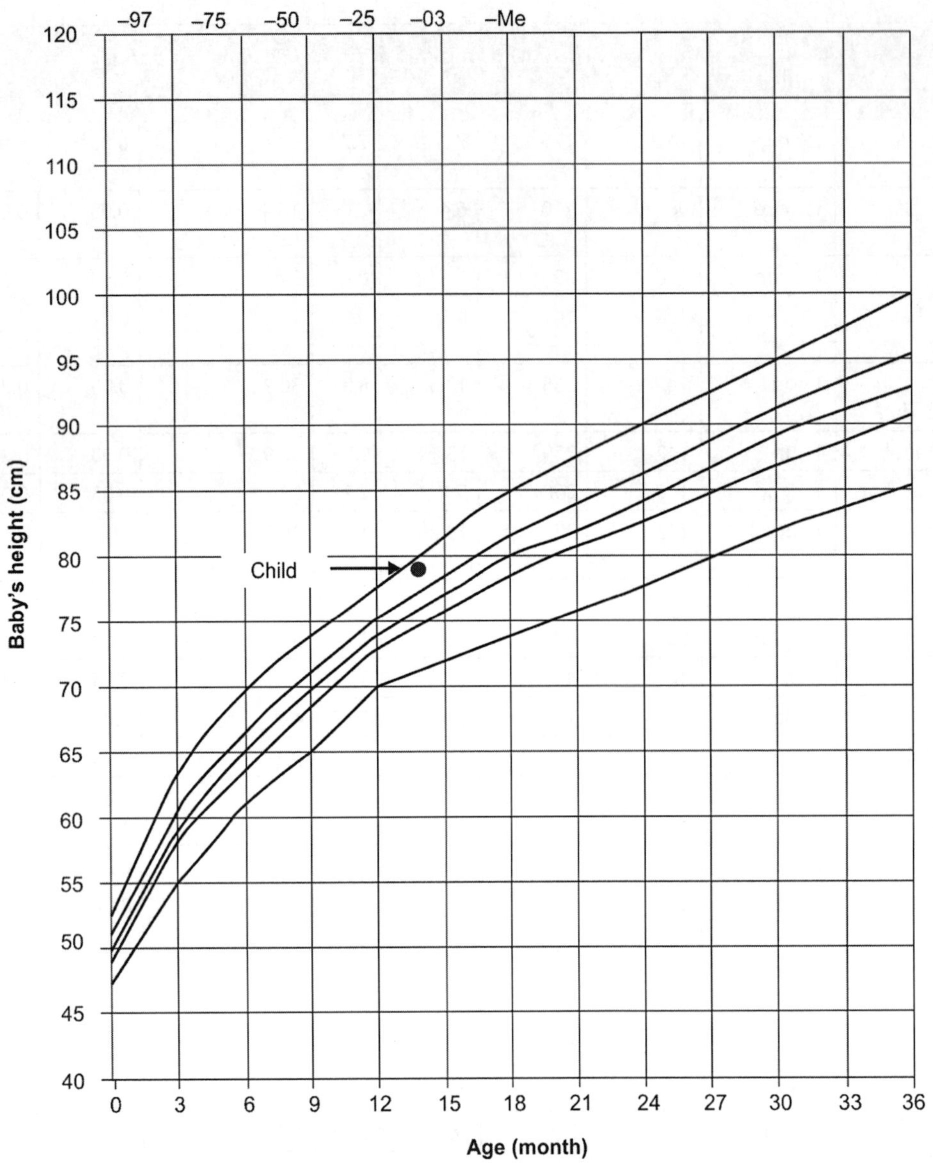

Figure 17.1: Baby's growth chart—height (0–36 month)

Nutritional Assessment for Under-five Children

Name of the village/area : ____________________

Name of the family head : ____________________

House number : ____________________

Particulars of Parents

Sl No.	Name of the parents	Age	Sex	Education	Occupation	Remarks
1.						
2.						
3.						

Number of living children : ____________________

Sl No.	Name of the children	Order of live birth	Date of birth	Age	Sex	Education
1.						
2.						
3.						

Anthropometric Measurement

Weight (kg) : ____________________

Height/Length (cm) : ____________________

Head circumference (cm) : ____________________

Chest circumference (cm) : ____________________

Mid-arm circumference (cm) : ____________________

Clinical Examination

General impression : ____________________

Apathy : ____________________

Pallor : ____________________

Ability : ____________________

Hair

Loss of luster : ____________________

Thinning : ____________________

Sparse : ____________________

Easily plucked : ____________________

Flag sign : ____________________

Face

Moon face : ____________________

Nasolabial dyssebacia : ____________________

Eyes

Pigmentation of conjunctiva : ____________________

Conjunctival necrosis : ____________________

Bitot's spot : ____________________

Corneal xerosis and keratomalacia : Normal/Hasy/Opaque

Night blindness : ____________________

Angular conjunctivitis : ____________________

False conjunctivitis : ____________________

Lips

Angular stomatitis : ____________________

Cheilosis : ____________________

Tongue

Red and raw : ____________________

Papilla (atrophic) : ____________________

Teeth

Caries : ____________________

Mottled enamel : ____________________

Gums

Spongy bleeding : ____________________

If any, specify : ____________________

Gland

Goiter : ____________________

If any, specify : ____________________

Skin

Follicular hyperkeratosis
(phrynoderma) : ____________________

Mosaic dermatosis : ____________________

Pellagrous dermatitis : ____________________

Crazy-pavement dermatosis : ____________________

Nail

Spooning of the nails : ______________________

Subcutaneous tissues

Edema : ______________________

Marasmus : ______________________

Skeletal system

Cranial bossing (frontal) : ______________________

Cranial bossing (parital) : ______________________

Craniotabes : ______________________

Beading of ribs : ______________________

Knock-knees/Bow legs : ______________________

Nervous system

Numbness and tingling of extremities : ______________________

Burning feet : ______________________

Tenderness of calf muscles : ______________________

Loss of knee/ankle/jerks : ______________________

Blood

Hemoglobin : ______________________

Clinical impression

Marasmus : ______________________

Prekwashiorkor : ______________________

Kwashiorkor : ______________________

Others (specify) : ______________________

List Out Nursing Diagnosis

1.
2.
3.
4.
5.
6.
7.

Nutritional Assessment of Under-five Children

Case 2

Name of the Village/Area : ________________

House Number : ________________

Name of the Family Head : ________________

Age/Sex : ________________

Educational Status : ________________

Occupational Status : ________________

Address : ________________

____

____

Common Cooking Method : Steaming/Boiling/Deep/Shallow frying

Preparation of Food : Hygienic/Unhygienic

Commonly Consuming Food Items : ________________

____

Particulars of Parents

Sl No.	Name of the parents	Age	Sex	Education	Occupation	Remarks
1.						
2.						

Number of living children : ________________

Sl No.	Name of the children	Order of live birth	Date of birth	Age	Sex	Education
1.						
2.						
3.						

Anthropometric Measurement

Weight (kg) : ________________

Height/Length (cm) : ________________

Head circumference (cm) : ________________

Chest circumference (cm) : ____________________

Mid-arm circumference (cm) : ____________________

Degree of Malnutrition

Body Mass Index

Growth Chart

24-hour Dietary Recall Survey

Name of the area : ____________________

Taluk : ____________________

District : ____________________

Religion : ____________________

Total number of family members : ____________________

Family income : ____________________

Family Characteristics

Sl No.	Name	Age	Occupation			Vegetarian	Nonvegetarian
			Sedentary	Moderate	Hard		
1.							
2.							
3.							
4.							
5.							
6.							

Purchase of Raw Material and their Expenditure Per Day

Items	How often purchasing?			Monthly	Seasonally	Quantity	Expenditure per day
	Daily	By weekly	Weekly				
Cereals							
Pulses							
Milk							
Fruits							
Vegetables							
Jaggery							
Sugar							
Ghee							
Oil							
Eggs							
Meat							
Fish							

Shopping facilities : Markets/Village shop/Stores/Any other forms
Preservation of raw foods : Store room/Kitchen/No store/Living room
Preservation of cooked food : Refrigerator/Cupboard/Kitchen
Fuel used for cooking : Cooking gas/Electrical stove/Firewood/Kerosene stove

Do you have:

Vegetable garden? ______

Fruit tree? ______

Household Animals

Cow : ______
Buffalo : ______
Hen : ______
Goat : ______
Pig : ______

Nutrition Cycle of the Family

Items/Days	Items in gram							Average daily intake	Category
	1	2	3	4	5	6	7		
Wheat									Cereals
Rice									
Jowar									
Bajara									
Other									
Toor dal									Pulses
Arhar									
Urad									
Moong									
Green gram									
Ground nuts									
Others									
Milk									Milk products
Curd									

Contd...

Contd...

Items/Days	Items in gram							Average daily intake	Category
	1	2	3	4	5	6	7		
Buttermilk									
Others									
Oil									Fats
Ghee									
Dalda									
Leafy vegetables									Vegetables
Root/Tubers									
Others									
Tea									Beverage
Coffee									
Others									
Sugar									Sweeteners
Jaggery									
Meat									Animals foods
Fish									
Egg									
Banana									Fruits
Orange									
Papaya									
Pineapple									
Grapes									
Apple									
Guava									
Others									

Inference

___

___

___

WHO recommended nutritive values for commonly used food items in India

Sl No.	Food preparation	Quantity per serving	Weight per serving	Calories (kcal)	Protein (g)	Fat (g)	Carbohydrates (g)	Calcium (g)	Phosphorus (g)	Iron (mg)
Cereal and millet preparation										
I	*Rice preparation*									
1.	Plain rice	2 serving	504	595	11.9	0.9	134.8	0.02	0.2	11.9
2.	Sambar rice	1 serving	485	405	13.5	13.5	76.2	0.08	0.16	13.5
3.	Curd rice	1 serving	253	221	6	7	33.3	0.57	0.10	6
4.	Sweet rice	1 serving	177	432	3.6	12	77.4	0.01	0.05	3.6
5.	Idli	2 pcs	136	130	4.6	0.2	27.6	0.03	0.08	4.6
6.	Plain dosa	2 pcs	100	216	4.1	9.7	28.2	0.03	0.07	4 1
7.	Masala dosa	2 pcs	100	212	4.6	8 4	29.4	0.04	0.08	4.6
8.	Pongal (hot)	1 serving	148	200	5.5	6	30.5	0.03	0.07	5.5
9.	Adai (hot)	1 pc	96	195	6.6	4.4	31.8	0.03	0.09	6.6
II	*Wheat preparation*									
1.	Wheat upma	1 serving	128	163	3.8	5.4	24.7	0.01	0.04	0.7
2.	Chapatis	2 pcs	57	196	5	5.5	30.8	0.13	0.02	3
3.	Puris	2 pcs	32	136	2.2	8.4	13	0.06	0.01	1.3
4.	Plain parathas	1 pc	66	104	4.5	19.6	27.3	0.12	0.01	2.7
5.	Rava (dosa, idli)	2 pcs	114	212	5	8.5	28.7	0	0.06	0.9
6.	Kesari bath	1 serving	90	284	2	14.6	35.3	0.02	0.04	0.44
7.	Luchi	2 pcs	71	346	4	24	28	0.03	0.01	0.4
III	*Millet preparation*									
1.	Ragi balls	1 pc	336	446	6	7.6	86.8	0.3	0.4	6
2.	Ragi roti	2 pcs	185	460	8	9	87	0.3	0.4	6
3.	Maize roti	2 pcs	142	314	9.6	5.5	56.4	0.3	0.1	1.8
4.	Jowar roti	2 pcs	150	252	7.5	1.3	52.5	0.2	0.02	4.5
5.	Ragi puttu	1 serving	146	422	4.4	7.4	84	0.2	0.02	
IV	*Pulse preparation*									
1.	Bengal gram dal (cooked)	1½ cup	157	284	9	16.4	25.2	0.07	0.13	3.8
2.	Bengal gram dal	1 cup	154	178	3.2	35.9	44.7	0.09	0.08	0.4

Contd...

Contd...

Sl No.	Food preparation	Quantity per serving	Weight per serving	Calories (kcal)	Protein (g)	Fat (g)	Carbohydrates (g)	Calcium (g)	Phosphorus (g)	Iron (mg)
3.	Green gram dal (cooked)	1½ cup	142	171	7	7.7	18.4	0.08	0.09	2.7
4.	Red gram dal (cooked)	1½ cup	96	110	6.4	2	16.4	0.05	0.07	2.6
5.	Dal rasam	1½ cup	196	29	1.5	0.9	3.8	0.03	0.03	0.09
6.	Radish sambar (sundal)		196	101	4.1	3.6	13.1	0.04	0.07	2.2
7.	Green gram sambar (sundal)	1 cup	142	255	13.5	8.8	30.3	0.05	0.2	2.5
8.	Cowpea sundal	1 cup	142	259	13.1	9.2	30.9	0.08	0.2	4.8
9.	Amaranth sambar	1½ cup	140	250	5.1	2.7	13	0.05	0.08	8
10.	Bengal gram (sundal)	1 cup	142	272	13.2	11.1	29.7	0.11	0.15	5.5
V	*Vegetable preparation*									
1.	Amaranth curry	1½ plate	28	47	1.4	2.3	5.1	0.04	0.04	6.64
2.	Amaranth masala	½ plate	42	46	1.2	2.6	4.4	0.05	0.05	6.8
3.	Brinjal curry	½ plate	45	122	1.4	10.7	4.9	0.02	0.05	0.9
4.	Milk (buffalo)	1 cup	200	216	8.4	16	9.2	0.42	0.030	0.8
5.	Cabbage and carrot curry	½ plate	56	81	1.5	5.6	6.1	0.04	0.12	0.9
6.	Buttermilk	1 cup	200	36	1.8	2.8	2	0.07	0.07	0.2
7.	Buttermilk (buffalo)	1 cup	200	66	24	5.4	2.8	0.07	0.07	0.2
VI	*Egg, milk and meat preparation*									
1.	Meat curry	1 serving	128	220	116	18	2.7	0.1	0.01	2.1
2.	Omelet	1 serving	39	77	5.8	5.7	0.5	0.03	0.1	1
3.	Meat fry	1 serving	142	339	21.8	26	4.5	0.23	0.2	3.3
4.	Fish fry	1 serving	100	220	16.2	16.2	1.4	0.05	0.45	1.2
5.	Rice, mutton pulao	2 servings	341	686	39	39	63.6	0.1	0.22	1.5
VII	*Preparation containing milk*									
1.	Coffee	1 cup	200	104	3.8	3.4	14.4	0.1	0.1	1.2
2.	Tea	1 cup	200	72	1.4	1.6	13	0.06	0.04	-
3.	Cocoa	1 cup	200	174	7.5	20.2	20.2	0.2	0.15	0.3
4.	Wheat payasam	1 cup	154	178	3.4	31.5	31.5	0.09	0.08	0.4
5.	Rice payasam	1 cup	266	227	3.7	44.3	44.3	0.14	0.1	4.7
6.	Rice porridge	1 cup	280	263	7.6	44.7	35.9	0.3	0.2	0.7
7.	Soy porridge	1 cup	154	178	7.7	44	44.7	0.07	0.14	0.4
8.	Wheat porridge	1 cup	280	263	7.6	44.7	35.9	0.3	0.22	0.7
9.	Ragi porridge	1 cup	193	317	8.7	52.7	35.9	0.24	0.22	1
10.	Milk (cow)	1 cup	200	130	7	9.8	52.7	0.12	0.1	0.4

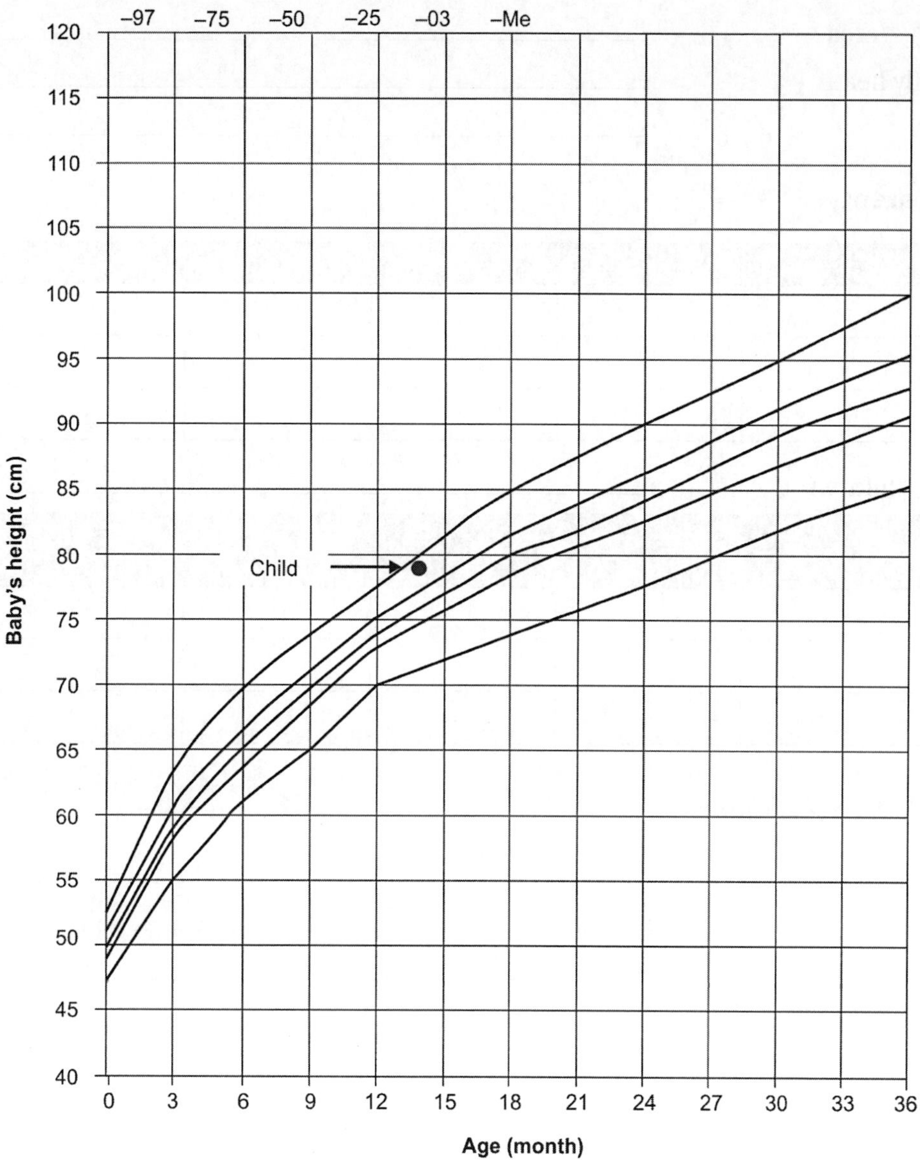

Figure 17.1: Baby's growth chart—height (0–36 month)

Nutritional Assessment for Under-five Children

Name of the village/area : __________

Name of the family head : __________

House number : __________

Particulars of Parents

Sl No.	Name of the parents	Age	Sex	Education	Occupation	Remarks
1.						
2.						
3.						

Number of living children : __________

Sl No.	Name of the children	Order of live birth	Date of birth	Age	Sex	Education
1.						
2.						
3.						

Anthropometric Measurement

Weight (kg) : __________

Height/Length (cm) : __________

Head circumference (cm) : __________

Chest circumference (cm) : __________

Mid-arm circumference (cm) : __________

Clinical Examination

General impression : __________

Apathy : __________

Pallor : __________

Ability : __________

Hair

Loss of luster : __________

Thinning : __________

Sparse : __________

Easily plucked : __________

Flag sign : ______

Face

Moon face : ______

Nasolabial dyssebacia : ______

Eyes

Pigmentation of conjunctiva : ______

Conjunctival necrosis : ______

Bitot's spot : ______

Corneal xerosis and keratomalacia : Normal/Hasy/Opaque

Night blindness : ______

Angular conjunctivitis : ______

False conjunctivitis : ______

Lips

Angular stomatitis : ______

Cheilosis : ______

Tongue

Red and raw : ______

Papilla (atrophic) : ______

Teeth

Caries : ______

Mottled enamel : ______

Gums

Spongy bleeding : ______

If any, specify : ______

Gland

Goiter : ______

If any, specify : ______

Skin

Follicular hyperkeratosis (phrynoderma) : ______

Mosaic dermatosis : ______

Pellagrous dermatitis : ______

Crazy-pavement dermatosis : ______

Nail

Spooning of the nails : ____________________

Subcutaneous tissues

Edema : ____________________

Marasmus : ____________________

Skeletal system

Cranial bossing (frontal) : ____________________

Cranial bossing (parital) : ____________________

Craniotabes : ____________________

Beading of ribs : ____________________

Knock-knees/Bow legs : ____________________

Nervous system

Numbness and tingling of extremities : ____________________

Burning feet : ____________________

Tenderness of calf muscles : ____________________

Loss of knee/ankle/jerks : ____________________

Blood

Hemoglobin : ____________________

Clinical impression

Marasmus : ____________________

Prekwashiorkor : ____________________

Kwashiorkor : ____________________

Others (specify) : ____________________

List Out Nursing Diagnosis

1.
2.
3.
4.
5.
6.
7.

Nutritional Assessment of Under-five Children

Case 3

Name of the Village/Area : ______________________

House Number : ______________________

Name of the Family Head : ______________________

Age/Sex : ______________________

Educational Status : ______________________

Occupational Status : ______________________

Address : ______________________

____

____

Common Cooking Method : Steaming/Boiling/Deep/Shallow frying

Preparation of Food : Hygienic/Unhygienic

Commonly Consuming Food Items : ______________________

____

Particulars of Parents

Sl No.	Name of the parents	Age	Sex	Education	Occupation	Remarks
1.						
2.						

Number of living children : ______________________

Sl No.	Name of the children	Order of live birth	Date of birth	Age	Sex	Education
1.						
2.						
3.						

Anthropometric Measurement

Weight (kg) : ______________________

Height/Length (cm) : ______________________

Head circumference (cm) : ______________________

Chest circumference (cm) : ______________________________

Mid-arm circumference (cm) : ______________________________

Degree of Malnutrition

____
____
____
____
____
____

Body Mass Index

____
____
____
____
____
____

Growth Chart

24-hour Dietary Recall Survey

Name of the area : ____________________

Taluk : ____________________

District : ____________________

Religion : ____________________

Total number of family members : ____________________

Family income : ____________________

Family Characteristics

Sl No.	Name	Age	Occupation			Vegetarian	Nonvegetarian
			Sedentary	Moderate	Hard		
1.							
2.							
3.							
4.							
5.							
6.							

Purchase of Raw Material and their Expenditure Per Day

Items	How often purchasing?			Monthly	Seasonally	Quantity	Expenditure per day
	Daily	By weekly	Weekly				
Cereals							
Pulses							
Milk							
Fruits							
Vegetables							
Jaggery							
Sugar							
Ghee							
Oil							
Eggs							
Meat							
Fish							

Shopping facilities : Markets/Village shop/Stores/Any other forms

Preservation of raw foods : Store room/Kitchen/No store/Living room

Preservation of cooked food : Refrigerator/Cupboard/Kitchen

Fuel used for cooking : Cooking gas/Electrical stove/Firewood/Kerosene stove

Do you have:

Vegetable garden? ______________________

Fruit tree? ______________________

Household Animals

Cow : ______________________

Buffalo : ______________________

Hen : ______________________

Goat : ______________________

Pig : ______________________

Nutrition Cycle of the Family

Items/Days	Items in gram							Average daily intake	Category
	1	2	3	4	5	6	7		
Wheat									Cereals
Rice									
Jowar									
Bajara									
Other									
Toor dal									Pulses
Arhar									
Urad									
Moong									
Green gram									
Ground nuts									
Others									
Milk									Milk products
Curd									

Contd...

Contd...

Items/Days	Items in gram							Average daily intake	Category
	1	2	3	4	5	6	7		
Buttermilk									
Others									
Oil									Fats
Ghee									
Dalda									
Leafy vegetables									Vegetables
Root/Tubers									
Others									
Tea									Beverage
Coffee									
Others									
Sugar									Sweeteners
Jaggery									
Meat									Animals foods
Fish									
Egg									
Banana									Fruits
Orange									
Papaya									
Pineapple									
Grapes									
Apple									
Guava									
Others									

Inference

____

____

____

WHO recommended nutritive values for commonly used food items in India

Sl No.	Food preparation	Quantity per serving	Weight per serving	Calories (kcal)	Protein (g)	Fat (g)	Carbohydrates (g)	Calcium (g)	Phosphorus (g)	Iron (mg)
Cereal and millet preparation										
I	*Rice preparation*									
1.	Plain rice	2 serving	504	595	11.9	0.9	134.8	0.02	0.2	11.9
2.	Sambar rice	1 serving	485	405	13.5	13.5	76.2	0.08	0.16	13.5
3.	Curd rice	1 serving	253	221	6	7	33.3	0.57	0.10	6
4.	Sweet rice	1 serving	177	432	3.6	12	77.4	0.01	0.05	3.6
5.	Idli	2 pcs	136	130	4.6	0.2	27.6	0.03	0.08	4.6
6.	Plain dosa	2 pcs	100	216	4.1	9.7	28.2	0.03	0.07	4 1
7.	Masala dosa	2 pcs	100	212	4.6	8 4	29.4	0.04	0.08	4.6
8.	Pongal (hot)	1 serving	148	200	5.5	6	30.5	0.03	0.07	5.5
9.	Adai (hot)	1 pc	96	195	6.6	4.4	31.8	0.03	0.09	6.6
II	*Wheat preparation*									
1.	Wheat upma	1 serving	128	163	3.8	5.4	24.7	0.01	0.04	0.7
2.	Chapatis	2 pcs	57	196	5	5.5	30.8	0.13	0.02	3
3.	Puris	2 pcs	32	136	2.2	8.4	13	0.06	0.01	1.3
4.	Plain parathas	1 pc	66	104	4.5	19.6	27.3	0.12	0.01	2.7
5.	Rava (dosa, idli)	2 pcs	114	212	5	8.5	28.7	0	0.06	0.9
6.	Kesari bath	1 serving	90	284	2	14.6	35.3	0.02	0.04	0.44
7.	Luchi	2 pcs	71	346	4	24	28	0.03	0.01	0.4
III	*Millet preparation*									
1.	Ragi balls	1 pc	336	446	6	7.6	86.8	0.3	0.4	6
2.	Ragi roti	2 pcs	185	460	8	9	87	0.3	0.4	6
3.	Maize roti	2 pcs	142	314	9.6	5.5	56.4	0.3	0.1	1.8
4.	Jowar roti	2 pcs	150	252	7.5	1.3	52.5	0.2	0.02	4.5
5.	Ragi puttu	1 serving	146	422	4.4	7.4	84	0.2	0.02	
IV	*Pulse preparation*									
1.	Bengal gram dal (cooked)	1½ cup	157	284	9	16.4	25.2	0.07	0.13	3.8
2.	Bengal gram dal	1 cup	154	178	3.2	35.9	44.7	0.09	0.08	0.4

Contd...

Contd...

Sl No.	Food preparation	Quantity per serving	Weight per serving	Calories (kcal)	Protein (g)	Fat (g)	Carbohydrates (g)	Calcium (g)	Phosphorus (g)	Iron (mg)
3.	Green gram dal (cooked)	1½ cup	142	171	7	7.7	18.4	0.08	0.09	2.7
4.	Red gram dal (cooked)	1½ cup	96	110	6.4	2	16.4	0.05	0.07	2.6
5.	Dal rasam	1½ cup	196	29	1.5	0.9	3.8	0.03	0.03	0.09
6.	Radish sambar (sundal)		196	101	4.1	3.6	13.1	0.04	0.07	2.2
7.	Green gram sambar (sundal)	1 cup	142	255	13.5	8.8	30.3	0.05	0.2	2.5
8.	Cowpea sundal	1 cup	142	259	13.1	9.2	30.9	0.08	0.2	4.8
9.	Amaranth sambar	1½ cup	140	250	5.1	2.7	13	0.05	0.08	8
10.	Bengal gram (sundal)	1 cup	142	272	13.2	11.1	29.7	0.11	0.15	5.5
V	*Vegetable preparation*									
1.	Amaranth curry	1½ plate	28	47	1.4	2.3	5.1	0.04	0.04	6.64
2.	Amaranth masala	½ plate	42	46	1.2	2.6	4.4	0.05	0.05	6.8
3.	Brinjal curry	½ plate	45	122	1.4	10.7	4.9	0.02	0.05	0.9
4.	Milk (buffalo)	1 cup	200	216	8.4	16	9.2	0.42	0.030	0.8
5.	Cabbage and carrot curry	½ plate	56	81	1.5	5.6	6.1	0.04	0.12	0.9
6.	Buttermilk	1 cup	200	36	1.8	2.8	2	0.07	0.07	0.2
7.	Buttermilk (buffalo)	1 cup	200	66	24	5.4	2.8	0.07	0.07	0.2
VI	*Egg, milk and meat preparation*									
1.	Meat curry	1 serving	128	220	116	18	2.7	0.1	0.01	2.1
2.	Omelet	1 serving	39	77	5.8	5.7	0.5	0.03	0.1	1
3.	Meat fry	1 serving	142	339	21.8	26	4.5	0.23	0.2	3.3
4.	Fish fry	1 serving	100	220	16.2	16.2	1.4	0.05	0.45	1.2
5.	Rice, mutton pulao	2 servings	341	686	39	39	63.6	0.1	0.22	1.5
VII	*Preparation containing milk*									
1.	Coffee	1 cup	200	104	3.8	3.4	14.4	0.1	0.1	1.2
2.	Tea	1 cup	200	72	1.4	1.6	13	0.06	0.04	-
3.	Cocoa	1 cup	200	174	7.5	20.2	20.2	0.2	0.15	0.3
4.	Wheat payasam	1 cup	154	178	3.4	31.5	31.5	0.09	0.08	0.4
5.	Rice payasam	1 cup	266	227	3.7	44.3	44.3	0.14	0.1	4.7
6.	Rice porridge	1 cup	280	263	7.6	44.7	35.9	0.3	0.2	0.7
7.	Soy porridge	1 cup	154	178	7.7	44	44.7	0.07	0.14	0.4
8.	Wheat porridge	1 cup	280	263	7.6	44.7	35.9	0.3	0.22	0.7
9.	Ragi porridge	1 cup	193	317	8.7	52.7	35.9	0.24	0.22	1
10.	Milk (cow)	1 cup	200	130	7	9.8	52.7	0.12	0.1	0.4

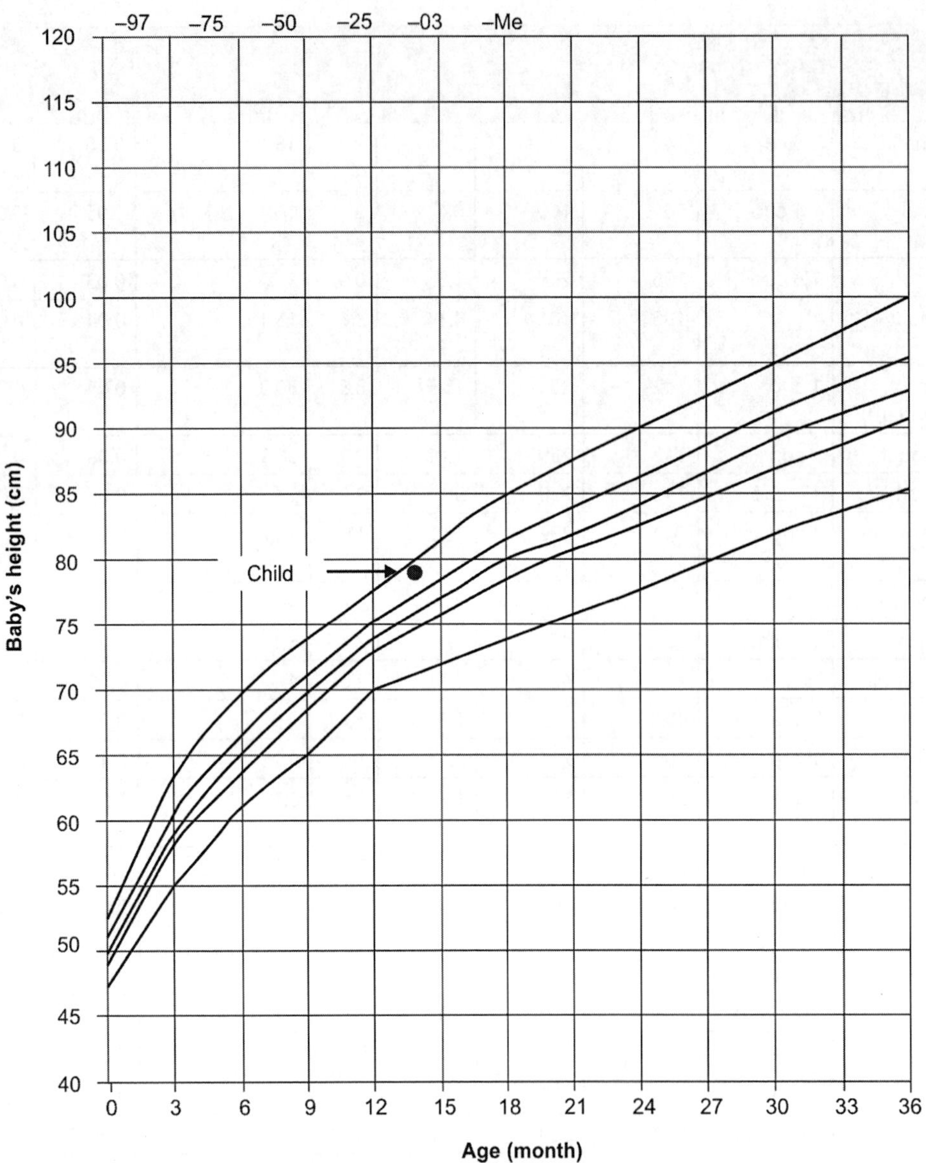

Figure 17.1: Baby's growth chart—height (0–36 month)

Nutritional Assessment for Under-five Children

Name of the village/area : __________
Name of the family head : __________
House number : __________

Particulars of Parents

Sl No.	Name of the parents	Age	Sex	Education	Occupation	Remarks
1.						
2.						
3.						

Number of living children : __________

Sl No.	Name of the children	Order of live birth	Date of birth	Age	Sex	Education
1.						
2.						
3.						

Anthropometric Measurement

Weight (kg) : __________
Height/Length (cm) : __________
Head circumference (cm) : __________
Chest circumference (cm) : __________
Mid-arm circumference (cm) : __________

Clinical Examination

General impression : __________
Apathy : __________
Pallor : __________
Ability : __________

Hair

Loss of luster : __________
Thinning : __________
Sparse : __________
Easily plucked : __________

Flag sign : ____________________

Face

Moon face : ____________________

Nasolabial dyssebacia : ____________________

Eyes

Pigmentation of conjunctiva : ____________________

Conjunctival necrosis : ____________________

Bitot's spot : ____________________

Corneal xerosis and keratomalacia : Normal/Hasy/Opaque

Night blindness : ____________________

Angular conjunctivitis : ____________________

False conjunctivitis : ____________________

Lips

Angular stomatitis : ____________________

Cheilosis : ____________________

Tongue

Red and raw : ____________________

Papilla (atrophic) : ____________________

Teeth

Caries : ____________________

Mottled enamel : ____________________

Gums

Spongy bleeding : ____________________

If any, specify : ____________________

Gland

Goiter : ____________________

If any, specify : ____________________

Skin

Follicular hyperkeratosis
(phrynoderma) : ____________________

Mosaic dermatosis : ____________________

Pellagrous dermatitis : ____________________

Crazy-pavement dermatosis : ____________________

Nail

Spooning of the nails : ______________________

Subcutaneous tissues

Edema : ______________________

Marasmus : ______________________

Skeletal system

Cranial bossing (frontal) : ______________________

Cranial bossing (parital) : ______________________

Craniotabes : ______________________

Beading of ribs : ______________________

Knock-knees/Bow legs : ______________________

Nervous system

Numbness and tingling of extremities : ______________________

Burning feet : ______________________

Tenderness of calf muscles : ______________________

Loss of knee/ankle/jerks : ______________________

Blood

Hemoglobin : ______________________

Clinical impression

Marasmus : ______________________

Prekwashiorkor : ______________________

Kwashiorkor : ______________________

Others (specify) : ______________________

List Out Nursing Diagnosis

1.
2.
3.
4.
5.
6.
7.

Nutritional Assessment of Under-five Children

Case 4

Name of the Village/Area : ____________________
House Number : ____________________
Name of the Family Head : ____________________
Age/Sex : ____________________
Educational Status : ____________________
Occupational Status : ____________________
Address : ____________________
____
____

Common Cooking Method : Steaming/Boiling/Deep/Shallow frying
Preparation of Food : Hygienic/Unhygienic
Commonly Consuming Food Items : ____________________
____

Particulars of Parents

Sl No.	Name of the parents	Age	Sex	Education	Occupation	Remarks
1.						
2.						

Number of living children : ____________________

Sl No.	Name of the children	Order of live birth	Date of birth	Age	Sex	Education
1.						
2.						
3.						

Anthropometric Measurement

Weight (kg) : ____________________
Height/Length (cm) : ____________________
Head circumference (cm) : ____________________

Chest circumference (cm) : ____________________
Mid-arm circumference (cm) : ____________________

Degree of Malnutrition

Body Mass Index

Growth Chart

24-hour Dietary Recall Survey

Name of the area : ______________________

Taluk : ______________________

District : ______________________

Religion : ______________________

Total number of family members : ______________________

Family income : ______________________

Family Characteristics

Sl No.	Name	Age	Occupation			Vegetarian	Nonvegetarian
			Sedentary	Moderate	Hard		
1.							
2.							
3.							
4.							
5.							
6.							

Purchase of Raw Material and their Expenditure Per Day

Items	How often purchasing?			Monthly	Seasonally	Quantity	Expenditure per day
	Daily	By weekly	Weekly				
Cereals							
Pulses							
Milk							
Fruits							
Vegetables							
Jaggery							
Sugar							
Ghee							
Oil							
Eggs							
Meat							
Fish							

Shopping facilities : Markets/Village shop/Stores/Any other forms
Preservation of raw foods : Store room/Kitchen/No store/Living room
Preservation of cooked food : Refrigerator/Cupboard/Kitchen
Fuel used for cooking : Cooking gas/Electrical stove/Firewood/Kerosene stove

Do you have:

Vegetable garden? ____________________

Fruit tree? ____________________

Household Animals

Cow : ____________________
Buffalo : ____________________
Hen : ____________________
Goat : ____________________
Pig : ____________________

Nutrition Cycle of the Family

Items/Days	Items in gram							Average daily intake	Category
	1	2	3	4	5	6	7		
Wheat									Cereals
Rice									
Jowar									
Bajara									
Other									
Toor dal									Pulses
Arhar									
Urad									
Moong									
Green gram									
Ground nuts									
Others									
Milk									Milk products
Curd									

Contd...

Contd...

Items/Days	Items in gram							Average daily intake	Category
	1	2	3	4	5	6	7		
Buttermilk									
Others									
Oil									Fats
Ghee									
Dalda									
Leafy vegetables									Vegetables
Root/Tubers									
Others									
Tea									Beverage
Coffee									
Others									
Sugar									Sweeteners
Jaggery									
Meat									Animals foods
Fish									
Egg									
Banana									Fruits
Orange									
Papaya									
Pineapple									
Grapes									
Apple									
Guava									
Others									

Inference

WHO recommended nutritive values for commonly used food items in India

Sl No.	Food preparation	Quantity per serving	Weight per serving	Calories (kcal)	Protein (g)	Fat (g)	Carbohydrates (g)	Calcium (g)	Phosphorus (g)	Iron (mg)
Cereal and millet preparation										
I	*Rice preparation*									
1.	Plain rice	2 serving	504	595	11.9	0.9	134.8	0.02	0.2	11.9
2.	Sambar rice	1 serving	485	405	13.5	13.5	76.2	0.08	0.16	13.5
3.	Curd rice	1 serving	253	221	6	7	33.3	0.57	0.10	6
4.	Sweet rice	1 serving	177	432	3.6	12	77.4	0.01	0.05	3.6
5.	Idli	2 pcs	136	130	4.6	0.2	27.6	0.03	0.08	4.6
6.	Plain dosa	2 pcs	100	216	4.1	9.7	28.2	0.03	0.07	4 1
7.	Masala dosa	2 pcs	100	212	4.6	8 4	29.4	0.04	0.08	4.6
8.	Pongal (hot)	1 serving	148	200	5.5	6	30.5	0.03	0.07	5.5
9.	Adai (hot)	1 pc	96	195	6.6	4.4	31.8	0.03	0.09	6.6
II	*Wheat preparation*									
1.	Wheat upma	1 serving	128	163	3.8	5.4	24.7	0.01	0.04	0.7
2.	Chapatis	2 pcs	57	196	5	5.5	30.8	0.13	0.02	3
3.	Puris	2 pcs	32	136	2.2	8.4	13	0.06	0.01	1.3
4.	Plain parathas	1 pc	66	104	4.5	19.6	27.3	0.12	0.01	2.7
5.	Rava (dosa, idli)	2 pcs	114	212	5	8.5	28.7	0	0.06	0.9
6.	Kesari bath	1 serving	90	284	2	14.6	35.3	0.02	0.04	0.44
7.	Luchi	2 pcs	71	346	4	24	28	0.03	0.01	0.4
III	*Millet preparation*									
1.	Ragi balls	1 pc	336	446	6	7.6	86.8	0.3	0.4	6
2.	Ragi roti	2 pcs	185	460	8	9	87	0.3	0.4	6
3.	Maize roti	2 pcs	142	314	9.6	5.5	56.4	0.3	0.1	1.8
4.	Jowar roti	2 pcs	150	252	7.5	1.3	52.5	0.2	0.02	4.5
5.	Ragi puttu	1 serving	146	422	4.4	7.4	84	0.2	0.02	
IV	*Pulse preparation*									
1.	Bengal gram dal (cooked)	1½ cup	157	284	9	16.4	25.2	0.07	0.13	3.8
2.	Bengal gram dal	1 cup	154	178	3.2	35.9	44.7	0.09	0.08	0.4

Contd...

Contd...

Sl No.	Food preparation	Quantity per serving	Weight per serving	Calories (kcal)	Protein (g)	Fat (g)	Carbohydrates (g)	Calcium (g)	Phosphorus (g)	Iron (mg)
3.	Green gram dal (cooked)	1½ cup	142	171	7	7.7	18.4	0.08	0.09	2.7
4.	Red gram dal (cooked)	1½ cup	96	110	6.4	2	16.4	0.05	0.07	2.6
5.	Dal rasam	1½ cup	196	29	1.5	0.9	3.8	0.03	0.03	0.09
6.	Radish sambar (sundal)		196	101	4.1	3.6	13.1	0.04	0.07	2.2
7.	Green gram sambar (sundal)	1 cup	142	255	13.5	8.8	30.3	0.05	0.2	2.5
8.	Cowpea sundal	1 cup	142	259	13.1	9.2	30.9	0.08	0.2	4.8
9.	Amaranth sambar	1½ cup	140	250	5.1	2.7	13	0.05	0.08	8
10.	Bengal gram (sundal)	1 cup	142	272	13.2	11.1	29.7	0.11	0.15	5.5
V	*Vegetable preparation*									
1.	Amaranth curry	1½ plate	28	47	1.4	2.3	5.1	0.04	0.04	6.64
2.	Amaranth masala	½ plate	42	46	1.2	2.6	4.4	0.05	0.05	6.8
3.	Brinjal curry	½ plate	45	122	1.4	10.7	4.9	0.02	0.05	0.9
4.	Milk (buffalo)	1 cup	200	216	8.4	16	9.2	0.42	0.030	0.8
5.	Cabbage and carrot curry	½ plate	56	81	1.5	5.6	6.1	0.04	0.12	0.9
6.	Buttermilk	1 cup	200	36	1.8	2.8	2	0.07	0.07	0.2
7.	Buttermilk (buffalo)	1 cup	200	66	24	5.4	2.8	0.07	0.07	0.2
VI	*Egg, milk and meat preparation*									
1.	Meat curry	1 serving	128	220	116	18	2.7	0.1	0.01	2.1
2.	Omelet	1 serving	39	77	5.8	5.7	0.5	0.03	0.1	1
3.	Meat fry	1 serving	142	339	21.8	26	4.5	0.23	0.2	3.3
4.	Fish fry	1 serving	100	220	16.2	16.2	1.4	0.05	0.45	1.2
5.	Rice, mutton pulao	2 servings	341	686	39	39	63.6	0.1	0.22	1.5
VII	*Preparation containing milk*									
1.	Coffee	1 cup	200	104	3.8	3.4	14.4	0.1	0.1	1.2
2.	Tea	1 cup	200	72	1.4	1.6	13	0.06	0.04	-
3.	Cocoa	1 cup	200	174	7.5	20.2	20.2	0.2	0.15	0.3
4.	Wheat payasam	1 cup	154	178	3.4	31.5	31.5	0.09	0.08	0.4
5.	Rice payasam	1 cup	266	227	3.7	44.3	44.3	0.14	0.1	4.7
6.	Rice porridge	1 cup	280	263	7.6	44.7	35.9	0.3	0.2	0.7
7.	Soy porridge	1 cup	154	178	7.7	44	44.7	0.07	0.14	0.4
8.	Wheat porridge	1 cup	280	263	7.6	44.7	35.9	0.3	0.22	0.7
9.	Ragi porridge	1 cup	193	317	8.7	52.7	35.9	0.24	0.22	1
10.	Milk (cow)	1 cup	200	130	7	9.8	52.7	0.12	0.1	0.4

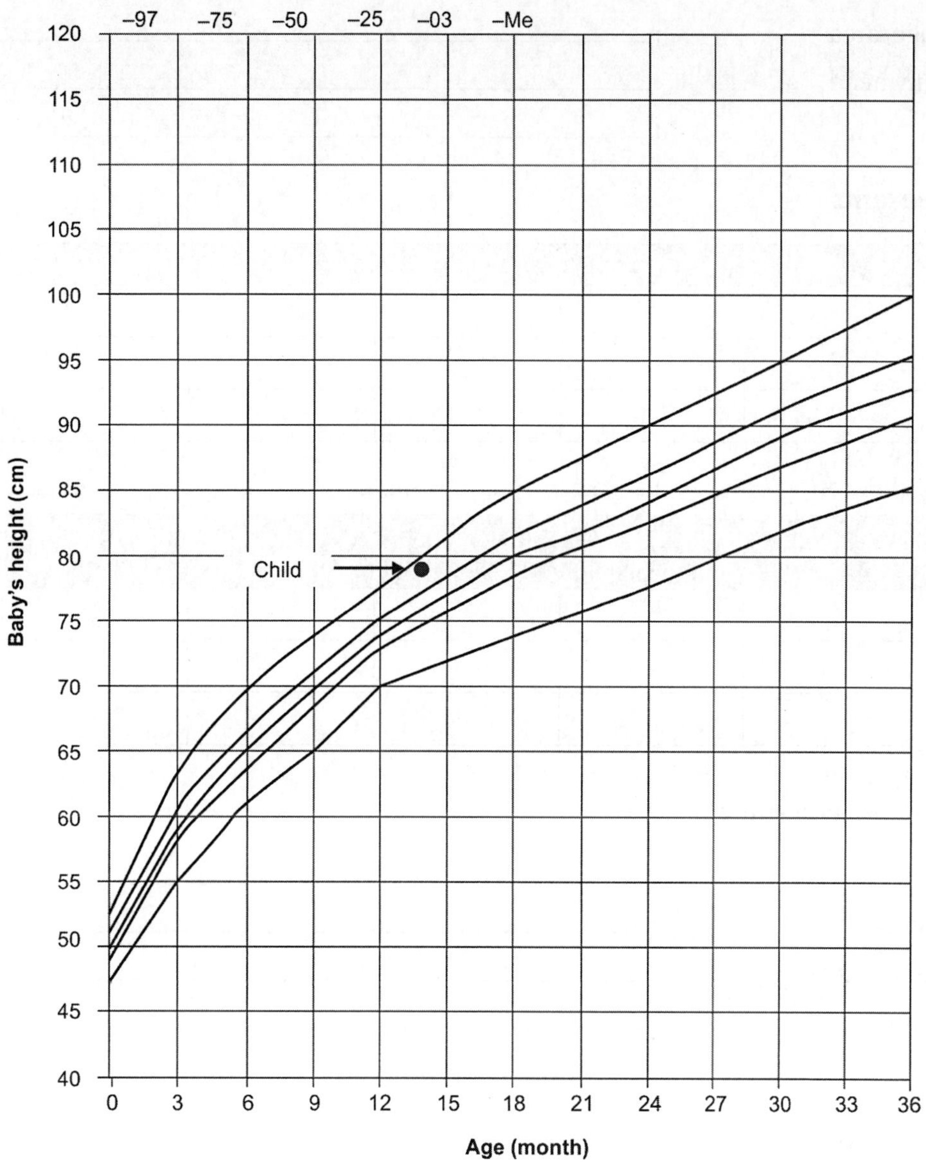

Figure 17.1: Baby's growth chart—height (0–36 month)

Nutritional Assessment for Under-five Children

Name of the village/area : ____________________

Name of the family head : ____________________

House number : ____________________

Particulars of Parents

Sl No.	Name of the parents	Age	Sex	Education	Occupation	Remarks
1.						
2.						
3.						

Number of living children : ____________________

Sl No.	Name of the children	Order of live birth	Date of birth	Age	Sex	Education
1.						
2.						
3.						

Anthropometric Measurement

Weight (kg) : ____________________

Height/Length (cm) : ____________________

Head circumference (cm) : ____________________

Chest circumference (cm) : ____________________

Mid-arm circumference (cm) : ____________________

Clinical Examination

General impression : ____________________

Apathy : ____________________

Pallor : ____________________

Ability : ____________________

Hair

Loss of luster : ____________________

Thinning : ____________________

Sparse : ____________________

Easily plucked : ____________________

Flag sign : ____________

Face

Moon face : ____________

Nasolabial dyssebacia : ____________

Eyes

Pigmentation of conjunctiva : ____________

Conjunctival necrosis : ____________

Bitot's spot : ____________

Corneal xerosis and keratomalacia : Normal/Hasy/Opaque

Night blindness : ____________

Angular conjunctivitis : ____________

False conjunctivitis : ____________

Lips

Angular stomatitis : ____________

Cheilosis : ____________

Tongue

Red and raw : ____________

Papilla (atrophic) : ____________

Teeth

Caries : ____________

Mottled enamel : ____________

Gums

Spongy bleeding : ____________

If any, specify : ____________

Gland

Goiter : ____________

If any, specify : ____________

Skin

Follicular hyperkeratosis
(phrynoderma) : ____________

Mosaic dermatosis : ____________

Pellagrous dermatitis : ____________

Crazy-pavement dermatosis : ____________

Nail

Spooning of the nails : __________

Subcutaneous tissues

Edema : __________

Marasmus : __________

Skeletal system

Cranial bossing (frontal) : __________

Cranial bossing (parital) : __________

Craniotabes : __________

Beading of ribs : __________

Knock-knees/Bow legs : __________

Nervous system

Numbness and tingling of extremities : __________

Burning feet : __________

Tenderness of calf muscles : __________

Loss of knee/ankle/jerks : __________

Blood

Hemoglobin : __________

Clinical impression

Marasmus : __________

Prekwashiorkor : __________

Kwashiorkor : __________

Others (specify) : __________

List Out Nursing Diagnosis

1.
2.
3.
4.
5.
6.
7.

Nutritional Assessment of Under-five Children

Case 5

Name of the Village/Area : ____________________

House Number : ____________________

Name of the Family Head : ____________________

Age/Sex : ____________________

Educational Status : ____________________

Occupational Status : ____________________

Address : ____________________

____

____

Common Cooking Method : Steaming/Boiling/Deep/Shallow frying

Preparation of Food : Hygienic/Unhygienic

Commonly Consuming Food Items : ____________________

____

Particulars of Parents

Sl No.	Name of the parents	Age	Sex	Education	Occupation	Remarks
1.						
2.						

Number of living children : ____________________

Sl No.	Name of the children	Order of live birth	Date of birth	Age	Sex	Education
1.						
2.						
3.						

Anthropometric Measurement

Weight (kg) : ____________________

Height/Length (cm) : ____________________

Head circumference (cm) : ____________________

Chest circumference (cm) : ____________________

Mid-arm circumference (cm) : ____________________

Degree of Malnutrition

____

____

____

____

____

____

Body Mass Index

____

____

____

____

____

____

Growth Chart

24-hour Dietary Recall Survey

Name of the area : ____________________

Taluk : ____________________

District : ____________________

Religion : ____________________

Total number of family members : ____________________

Family income : ____________________

Family Characteristics

Sl No.	Name	Age	Occupation			Vegetarian	Nonvegetarian
			Sedentary	Moderate	Hard		
1.							
2.							
3.							
4.							
5.							
6.							

Purchase of Raw Material and their Expenditure Per Day

Items	How often purchasing?			Monthly	Seasonally	Quantity	Expenditure per day
	Daily	By weekly	Weekly				
Cereals							
Pulses							
Milk							
Fruits							
Vegetables							
Jaggery							
Sugar							
Ghee							
Oil							
Eggs							
Meat							
Fish							

Shopping facilities : Markets/Village shop/Stores/Any other forms

Preservation of raw foods : Store room/Kitchen/No store/Living room

Preservation of cooked food : Refrigerator/Cupboard/Kitchen

Fuel used for cooking : Cooking gas/Electrical stove/Firewood/Kerosene stove

Do you have:

Vegetable garden? ____________________

Fruit tree? ____________________

Household Animals

Cow : ____________________

Buffalo : ____________________

Hen : ____________________

Goat : ____________________

Pig : ____________________

Nutrition Cycle of the Family

Items/Days	Items in gram							Average daily intake	Category
	1	2	3	4	5	6	7		
Wheat									Cereals
Rice									
Jowar									
Bajara									
Other									
Toor dal									Pulses
Arhar									
Urad									
Moong									
Green gram									
Ground nuts									
Others									
Milk									Milk products
Curd									

Contd...

Contd...

Items/Days	Items in gram							Average daily intake	Category
	1	2	3	4	5	6	7		
Buttermilk									
Others									
Oil									Fats
Ghee									
Dalda									
Leafy vegetables									Vegetables
Root/Tubers									
Others									
Tea									Beverage
Coffee									
Others									
Sugar									Sweeteners
Jaggery									
Meat									Animals foods
Fish									
Egg									
Banana									Fruits
Orange									
Papaya									
Pineapple									
Grapes									
Apple									
Guava									
Others									

Inference

____

____

____

WHO recommended nutritive values for commonly used food items in India

Sl No.	Food preparation	Quantity per serving	Weight per serving	Calories (kcal)	Protein (g)	Fat (g)	Carbohydrates (g)	Calcium (g)	Phosphorus (g)	Iron (mg)
Cereal and millet preparation										
I	*Rice preparation*									
1.	Plain rice	2 serving	504	595	11.9	0.9	134.8	0.02	0.2	11.9
2.	Sambar rice	1 serving	485	405	13.5	13.5	76.2	0.08	0.16	13.5
3.	Curd rice	1 serving	253	221	6	7	33.3	0.57	0.10	6
4.	Sweet rice	1 serving	177	432	3.6	12	77.4	0.01	0.05	3.6
5.	Idli	2 pcs	136	130	4.6	0.2	27.6	0.03	0.08	4.6
6.	Plain dosa	2 pcs	100	216	4.1	9.7	28.2	0.03	0.07	4 1
7.	Masala dosa	2 pcs	100	212	4.6	8 4	29.4	0.04	0.08	4.6
8.	Pongal (hot)	1 serving	148	200	5.5	6	30.5	0.03	0.07	5.5
9.	Adai (hot)	1 pc	96	195	6.6	4.4	31.8	0.03	0.09	6.6
II	*Wheat preparation*									
1.	Wheat upma	1 serving	128	163	3.8	5.4	24.7	0.01	0.04	0.7
2.	Chapatis	2 pcs	57	196	5	5.5	30.8	0.13	0.02	3
3.	Puris	2 pcs	32	136	2.2	8.4	13	0.06	0.01	1.3
4.	Plain parathas	1 pc	66	104	4.5	19.6	27.3	0.12	0.01	2.7
5.	Rava (dosa, idli)	2 pcs	114	212	5	8.5	28.7	0	0.06	0.9
6.	Kesari bath	1 serving	90	284	2	14.6	35.3	0.02	0.04	0.44
7.	Luchi	2 pcs	71	346	4	24	28	0.03	0.01	0.4
III	*Millet preparation*									
1.	Ragi balls	1 pc	336	446	6	7.6	86.8	0.3	0.4	6
2.	Ragi roti	2 pcs	185	460	8	9	87	0.3	0.4	6
3.	Maize roti	2 pcs	142	314	9.6	5.5	56.4	0.3	0.1	1.8
4.	Jowar roti	2 pcs	150	252	7.5	1.3	52.5	0.2	0.02	4.5
5.	Ragi puttu	1 serving	146	422	4.4	7.4	84	0.2	0.02	
IV	*Pulse preparation*									
1.	Bengal gram dal (cooked)	1½ cup	157	284	9	16.4	25.2	0.07	0.13	3.8
2.	Bengal gram dal	1 cup	154	178	3.2	35.9	44.7	0.09	0.08	0.4

Contd...

Contd...

Sl No.	Food preparation	Quantity per serving	Weight per serving	Calories (kcal)	Protein (g)	Fat (g)	Carbohydrates (g)	Calcium (g)	Phosphorus (g)	Iron (mg)
3.	Green gram dal (cooked)	1½ cup	142	171	7	7.7	18.4	0.08	0.09	2.7
4.	Red gram dal (cooked)	1½ cup	96	110	6.4	2	16.4	0.05	0.07	2.6
5.	Dal rasam	1½ cup	196	29	1.5	0.9	3.8	0.03	0.03	0.09
6.	Radish sambar (sundal)		196	101	4.1	3.6	13.1	0.04	0.07	2.2
7.	Green gram sambar (sundal)	1 cup	142	255	13.5	8.8	30.3	0.05	0.2	2.5
8.	Cowpea sundal	1 cup	142	259	13.1	9.2	30.9	0.08	0.2	4.8
9.	Amaranth sambar	1½ cup	140	250	5.1	2.7	13	0.05	0.08	8
10.	Bengal gram (sundal)	1 cup	142	272	13.2	11.1	29.7	0.11	0.15	5.5
V	*Vegetable preparation*									
1.	Amaranth curry	1½ plate	28	47	1.4	2.3	5.1	0.04	0.04	6.64
2.	Amaranth masala	½ plate	42	46	1.2	2.6	4.4	0.05	0.05	6.8
3.	Brinjal curry	½ plate	45	122	1.4	10.7	4.9	0.02	0.05	0.9
4.	Milk (buffalo)	1 cup	200	216	8.4	16	9.2	0.42	0.030	0.8
5.	Cabbage and carrot curry	½ plate	56	81	1.5	5.6	6.1	0.04	0.12	0.9
6.	Buttermilk	1 cup	200	36	1.8	2.8	2	0.07	0.07	0.2
7.	Buttermilk (buffalo)	1 cup	200	66	24	5.4	2.8	0.07	0.07	0.2
VI	*Egg, milk and meat preparation*									
1.	Meat curry	1 serving	128	220	116	18	2.7	0.1	0.01	2.1
2.	Omelet	1 serving	39	77	5.8	5.7	0.5	0.03	0.1	1
3.	Meat fry	1 serving	142	339	21.8	26	4.5	0.23	0.2	3.3
4.	Fish fry	1 serving	100	220	16.2	16.2	1.4	0.05	0.45	1.2
5.	Rice, mutton pulao	2 servings	341	686	39	39	63.6	0.1	0.22	1.5
VII	*Preparation containing milk*									
1.	Coffee	1 cup	200	104	3.8	3.4	14.4	0.1	0.1	1.2
2.	Tea	1 cup	200	72	1.4	1.6	13	0.06	0.04	-
3.	Cocoa	1 cup	200	174	7.5	20.2	20.2	0.2	0.15	0.3
4.	Wheat payasam	1 cup	154	178	3.4	31.5	31.5	0.09	0.08	0.4
5.	Rice payasam	1 cup	266	227	3.7	44.3	44.3	0.14	0.1	4.7
6.	Rice porridge	1 cup	280	263	7.6	44.7	35.9	0.3	0.2	0.7
7.	Soy porridge	1 cup	154	178	7.7	44	44.7	0.07	0.14	0.4
8.	Wheat porridge	1 cup	280	263	7.6	44.7	35.9	0.3	0.22	0.7
9.	Ragi porridge	1 cup	193	317	8.7	52.7	35.9	0.24	0.22	1
10.	Milk (cow)	1 cup	200	130	7	9.8	52.7	0.12	0.1	0.4

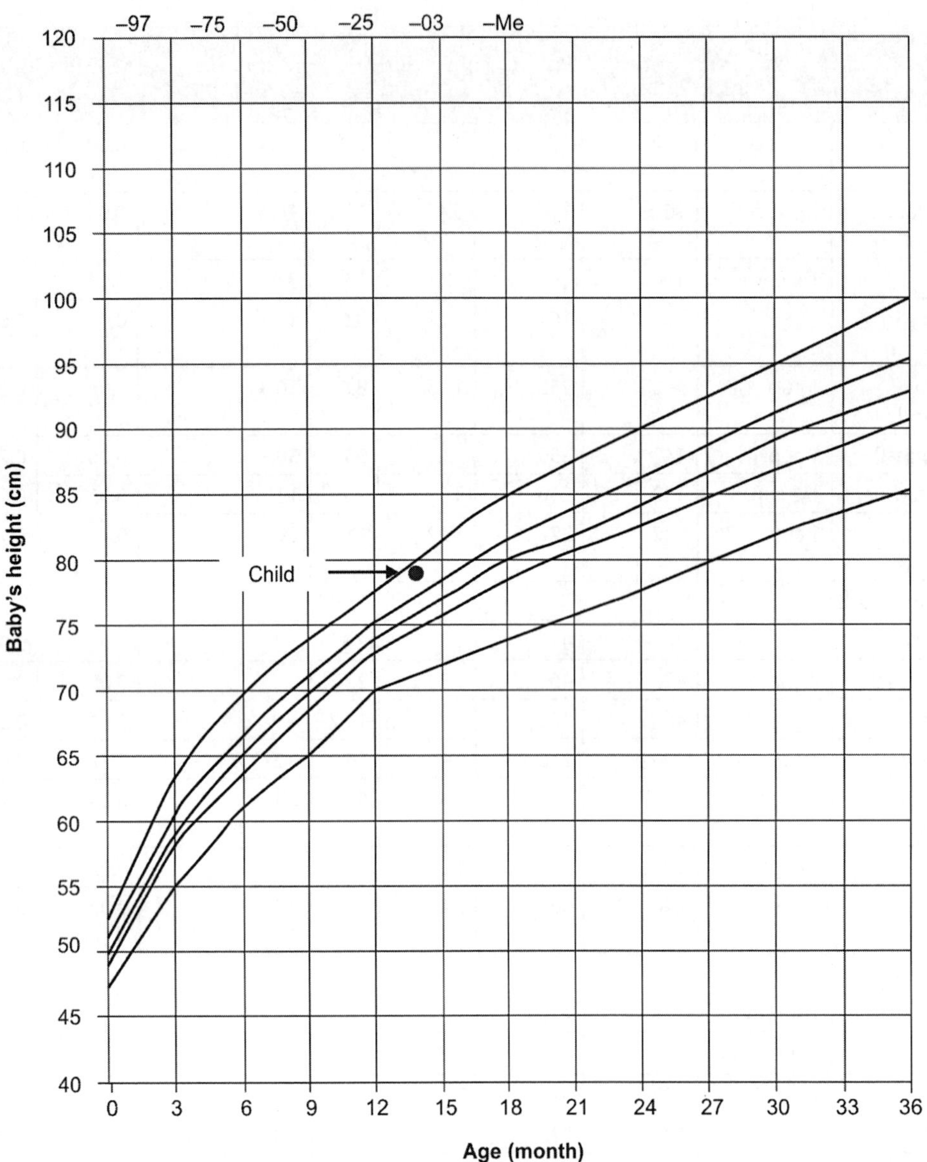

Figure 17.1: Baby's growth chart—height (0–36 month)

Nutritional Assessment for Under-five Children

Name of the village/area : ____________

Name of the family head : ____________

House number : ____________

Particulars of Parents

Sl No.	Name of the parents	Age	Sex	Education	Occupation	Remarks
1.						
2.						
3.						

Number of living children : ____________

Sl No.	Name of the children	Order of live birth	Date of birth	Age	Sex	Education
1.						
2.						
3.						

Anthropometric Measurement

Weight (kg) : ____________

Height/Length (cm) : ____________

Head circumference (cm) : ____________

Chest circumference (cm) : ____________

Mid-arm circumference (cm) : ____________

Clinical Examination

General impression : ____________

Apathy : ____________

Pallor : ____________

Ability : ____________

Hair

Loss of luster : ____________

Thinning : ____________

Sparse : ____________

Easily plucked : ____________

Flag sign : ______

Face

Moon face : ______

Nasolabial dyssebacia : ______

Eyes

Pigmentation of conjunctiva : ______

Conjunctival necrosis : ______

Bitot's spot : ______

Corneal xerosis and keratomalacia : Normal/Hasy/Opaque

Night blindness : ______

Angular conjunctivitis : ______

False conjunctivitis : ______

Lips

Angular stomatitis : ______

Cheilosis : ______

Tongue

Red and raw : ______

Papilla (atrophic) : ______

Teeth

Caries : ______

Mottled enamel : ______

Gums

Spongy bleeding : ______

If any, specify : ______

Gland

Goiter : ______

If any, specify : ______

Skin

Follicular hyperkeratosis (phrynoderma) : ______

Mosaic dermatosis : ______

Pellagrous dermatitis : ______

Crazy-pavement dermatosis : ______

Nail

Spooning of the nails : ____________________

Subcutaneous tissues

Edema : ____________________

Marasmus : ____________________

Skeletal system

Cranial bossing (frontal) : ____________________

Cranial bossing (parital) : ____________________

Craniotabes : ____________________

Beading of ribs : ____________________

Knock-knees/Bow legs : ____________________

Nervous system

Numbness and tingling of extremities : ____________________

Burning feet : ____________________

Tenderness of calf muscles : ____________________

Loss of knee/ankle/jerks : ____________________

Blood

Hemoglobin : ____________________

Clinical impression

Marasmus : ____________________

Prekwashiorkor : ____________________

Kwashiorkor : ____________________

Others (specify) : ____________________

List Out Nursing Diagnosis

1.
2.
3.
4.
5.
6.
7.

Cooking Demonstration

Case 1

Introduction

Purpose of Demonstration

Method of Cooking

Nutrition Values of Food

Items	Nutrient content	Amount of content	Nutrient value	Total value (calories)

WHO recommended nutritive values for commonly used food items in India

Sl No.	Food preparation	Quantity per serving	Weight per serving	Calories (kcal)	Protein (g)	Fat (g)	Carbohydrates (g)	Calcium (g)	Phosphorus (g)	Iron (mg)
Cereal and millet preparation										
I	*Rice preparation*									
1.	Plain rice	2 serving	504	595	11.9	0.9	134.8	0.02	0.2	11.9
2.	Sambar rice	1 serving	485	405	13.5	13.5	76.2	0.08	0.16	13.5
3.	Curd rice	1 serving	253	221	6	7	33.3	0.57	0.10	6
4.	Sweet rice	1 serving	177	432	3.6	12	77.4	0.01	0.05	3.6
5.	Idli	2 pcs	136	130	4.6	0.2	27.6	0.03	0.08	4.6
6.	Plain dosa	2 pcs	100	216	4.1	9.7	28.2	0.03	0.07	4 1
7.	Masala dosa	2 pcs	100	212	4.6	8 4	29.4	0.04	0.08	4.6
8.	Pongal (hot)	1 serving	148	200	5.5	6	30.5	0.03	0.07	5.5
9.	Adai (hot)	1 pc	96	195	6.6	4.4	31.8	0.03	0.09	6.6
II	*Wheat preparation*									
1.	Wheat upma	1 serving	128	163	3.8	5.4	24.7	0.01	0.04	0.7
2.	Chapatis	2 pcs	57	196	5	5.5	30.8	0.13	0.02	3
3.	Puris	2 pcs	32	136	2.2	8.4	13	0.06	0.01	1.3
4.	Plain parathas	1 pc	66	104	4.5	19.6	27.3	0.12	0.01	2.7
5.	Rava (dosa, idli)	2 pcs	114	212	5	8.5	28.7	0	0.06	0.9
6.	Kesari bath	1 serving	90	284	2	14.6	35.3	0.02	0.04	0.44
7.	Luchi	2 pcs	71	346	4	24	28	0.03	0.01	0.4
III	*Millet preparation*									
1.	Ragi balls	1 pc	336	446	6	7.6	86.8	0.3	0.4	6
2.	Ragi roti	2 pcs	185	460	8	9	87	0.3	0.4	6
3.	Maize roti	2 pcs	142	314	9.6	5.5	56.4	0.3	0.1	1.8
4.	Jowar roti	2 pcs	150	252	7.5	1.3	52.5	0.2	0.02	4.5
5.	Ragi puttu	1 serving	146	422	4.4	7.4	84	0.2	0.02	
IV	*Pulse preparation*									
1.	Bengal gram dal (cooked)	1½ cup	157	284	9	16.4	25.2	0.07	0.13	3.8
2.	Bengal gram dal	1 cup	154	178	3.2	35.9	44.7	0.09	0.08	0.4
3.	Green gram dal (cooked)	1½ cup	142	171	7	7.7	18.4	0.08	0.09	2.7
4.	Red gram dal (cooked)	1½ cup	96	110	6.4	2	16.4	0.05	0.07	2.6
5.	Dal rasam	1½ cup	196	29	1.5	0.9	3.8	0.03	0.03	0.09
6.	Radish sambar (sundal)		196	101	4.1	3.6	13.1	0.04	0.07	2.2
7.	Green gram sambar (sundal)	1 cup	142	255	13.5	8.8	30.3	0.05	0.2	2.5

Contd...

Contd...

Sl No.	Food preparation	Quantity per serving	Weight per serving	Calories (kcal)	Protein (g)	Fat (g)	Carbohydrates (g)	Calcium (g)	Phosphorus (g)	Iron (mg)
8.	Cowpea sundal	1 cup	142	259	13.1	9.2	30.9	0.08	0.2	4.8
9.	Amaranth sambar	1½ cup	140	250	5.1	2.7	13	0.05	0.08	8
10.	Bengal gram (sundal)	1 cup	142	272	13.2	11.1	29.7	0.11	0.15	5.5
V	*Vegetable preparation*									
1.	Amaranth curry	1½ plate	28	47	1.4	2.3	5.1	0.04	0.04	6.64
2.	Amaranth masala	½ plate	42	46	1.2	2.6	4.4	0.05	0.05	6.8
3.	Brinjal curry	½ plate	45	122	1.4	10.7	4.9	0.02	0.05	0.9
4.	Milk (buffalo)	1 cup	200	216	8.4	16	9.2	0.42	0.030	0.8
5.	Cabbage and carrot curry	½ plate	56	81	1.5	5.6	6.1	0.04	0.12	0.9
6.	Buttermilk	1 cup	200	36	1.8	2.8	2	0.07	0.07	0.2
7.	Buttermilk (buffalo)	1 cup	200	66	24	5.4	2.8	0.07	0.07	0.2
VI	*Egg, milk and meat preparation*									
1.	Meat curry	1 serving	128	220	116	18	2.7	0.1	0.01	2.1
2.	Omelet	1 serving	39	77	5.8	5.7	0.5	0.03	0.1	1
3.	Meat fry	1 serving	142	339	21.8	26	4.5	0.23	0.2	3.3
4.	Fish fry	1 serving	100	220	16.2	16.2	1.4	0.05	0.45	1.2
5.	Rice, mutton pulao	2 servings	341	686	39	39	63.6	0.1	0.22	1.5
VII	*Preparation containing milk*									
1.	Coffee	1 cup	200	104	3.8	3.4	14.4	0.1	0.1	1.2
2.	Tea	1 cup	200	72	1.4	1.6	13	0.06	0.04	-
3.	Cocoa	1 cup	200	174	7.5	20.2	20.2	0.2	0.15	0.3
4.	Wheat payasam	1 cup	154	178	3.4	31.5	31.5	0.09	0.08	0.4
5.	Rice payasam	1 cup	266	227	3.7	44.3	44.3	0.14	0.1	4.7
6.	Rice porridge	1 cup	280	263	7.6	44.7	35.9	0.3	0.2	0.7
7.	Soy porridge	1 cup	154	178	7.7	44	44.7	0.07	0.14	0.4
8.	Wheat porridge	1 cup	280	263	7.6	44.7	35.9	0.3	0.22	0.7
9.	Ragi porridge	1 cup	193	317	8.7	52.7	35.9	0.24	0.22	1
10.	Milk (cow)	1 cup	200	130	7	9.8	52.7	0.12	0.1	0.4

Health education regarding importance of nutrition

Time	Goals/Objectives	Activities		Audiovisual (AV) aids	Method of teaching	Evaluation
		Teacher	Client			

Contd...

Contd...

Time	Goals/Objectives	Activities		Audiovisual (AV) aids	Method of teaching	Evaluation
		Teacher	Client			

Contd...

Contd...

Time	Goals/Objectives	Activities		Audiovisual (AV) aids	Method of teaching	Evaluation
		Teacher	Client			

Contd...

Contd...

Time	Goals/Objectives	Activities		Audiovisual (AV) aids	Method of teaching	Evaluation
		Teacher	Client			

Contd...

Contd...

Time	Goals/Objectives	Activities		Audiovisual (AV) aids	Method of teaching	Evaluation
		Teacher	Client			

Evaluation for Cooking Demonstration

Name of the student : ______________________________

Batch (year) : ______________________________

Name of the recipient : ______________________________

Communication area : ______________________________

Date and time : ______________________________

Sl No.	Criteria	Marks allotted	Marks obtained
1.	Required item to be selected according to the needs of recipe	2	
2.	Prepared and summated on the time	2	
3.	Assessment of nutrition status of family	2	
4.	Family members interest	2	
5.	Way of preparation (hygiene, neat manner)	2	
6.	Selection of place and vessels	2	
7.	Way of serving	2	
8.	Cost benefit	2	
9.	Calculation of nutritive values for food items	2	
10.	Feedback from the family members	2	
	Total	**20**	

Signature of the Student
Date:

Signature of the Clinical Coordinator
Date:

Signature of the HOD of Community Health Nursing
Date:

Cooking Demonstration

Case 2

Introduction

Purpose of Demonstration

Method of Cooking

Nutrition Values of Food

Items	Nutrient content	Amount of content	Nutrient value	Total value (calories)

WHO recommended nutritive values for commonly used food items in India

Sl No.	Food preparation	Quantity per serving	Weight per serving	Calories (kcal)	Protein (g)	Fat (g)	Carbohydrates (g)	Calcium (g)	Phosphorus (g)	Iron (mg)
Cereal and millet preparation										
I	*Rice preparation*									
1.	Plain rice	2 serving	504	595	11.9	0.9	134.8	0.02	0.2	11.9
2.	Sambar rice	1 serving	485	405	13.5	13.5	76.2	0.08	0.16	13.5
3.	Curd rice	1 serving	253	221	6	7	33.3	0.57	0.10	6
4.	Sweet rice	1 serving	177	432	3.6	12	77.4	0.01	0.05	3.6
5.	Idli	2 pcs	136	130	4.6	0.2	27.6	0.03	0.08	4.6
6.	Plain dosa	2 pcs	100	216	4.1	9.7	28.2	0.03	0.07	4 1
7.	Masala dosa	2 pcs	100	212	4.6	8 4	29.4	0.04	0.08	4.6
8.	Pongal (hot)	1 serving	148	200	5.5	6	30.5	0.03	0.07	5.5
9.	Adai (hot)	1 pc	96	195	6.6	4.4	31.8	0.03	0.09	6.6
II	*Wheat preparation*									
1.	Wheat upma	1 serving	128	163	3.8	5.4	24.7	0.01	0.04	0.7
2.	Chapatis	2 pcs	57	196	5	5.5	30.8	0.13	0.02	3
3.	Puris	2 pcs	32	136	2.2	8.4	13	0.06	0.01	1.3
4.	Plain parathas	1 pc	66	104	4.5	19.6	27.3	0.12	0.01	2.7
5.	Rava (dosa, idli)	2 pcs	114	212	5	8.5	28.7	0	0.06	0.9
6.	Kesari bath	1 serving	90	284	2	14.6	35.3	0.02	0.04	0.44
7.	Luchi	2 pcs	71	346	4	24	28	0.03	0.01	0.4
III	*Millet preparation*									
1.	Ragi balls	1 pc	336	446	6	7.6	86.8	0.3	0.4	6
2.	Ragi roti	2 pcs	185	460	8	9	87	0.3	0.4	6
3.	Maize roti	2 pcs	142	314	9.6	5.5	56.4	0.3	0.1	1.8
4.	Jowar roti	2 pcs	150	252	7.5	1.3	52.5	0.2	0.02	4.5
5.	Ragi puttu	1 serving	146	422	4.4	7.4	84	0.2	0.02	
IV	*Pulse preparation*									
1.	Bengal gram dal (cooked)	1½ cup	157	284	9	16.4	25.2	0.07	0.13	3.8
2.	Bengal gram dal	1 cup	154	178	3.2	35.9	44.7	0.09	0.08	0.4
3.	Green gram dal (cooked)	1½ cup	142	171	7	7.7	18.4	0.08	0.09	2.7
4.	Red gram dal (cooked)	1½ cup	96	110	6.4	2	16.4	0.05	0.07	2.6
5.	Dal rasam	1½ cup	196	29	1.5	0.9	3.8	0.03	0.03	0.09
6.	Radish sambar (sundal)		196	101	4.1	3.6	13.1	0.04	0.07	2.2
7.	Green gram sambar (sundal)	1 cup	142	255	13.5	8.8	30.3	0.05	0.2	2.5

Contd...

Contd...

Sl No.	Food preparation	Quantity per serving	Weight per serving	Calories (kcal)	Protein (g)	Fat (g)	Carbohydrates (g)	Calcium (g)	Phosphorus (g)	Iron (mg)
8.	Cowpea sundal	1 cup	142	259	13.1	9.2	30.9	0.08	0.2	4.8
9.	Amaranth sambar	1½ cup	140	250	5.1	2.7	13	0.05	0.08	8
10.	Bengal gram (sundal)	1 cup	142	272	13.2	11.1	29.7	0.11	0.15	5.5
V	*Vegetable preparation*									
1.	Amaranth curry	1½ plate	28	47	1.4	2.3	5.1	0.04	0.04	6.64
2.	Amaranth masala	½ plate	42	46	1.2	2.6	4.4	0.05	0.05	6.8
3.	Brinjal curry	½ plate	45	122	1.4	10.7	4.9	0.02	0.05	0.9
4.	Milk (buffalo)	1 cup	200	216	8.4	16	9.2	0.42	0.030	0.8
5.	Cabbage and carrot curry	½ plate	56	81	1.5	5.6	6.1	0.04	0.12	0.9
6.	Buttermilk	1 cup	200	36	1.8	2.8	2	0.07	0.07	0.2
7.	Buttermilk (buffalo)	1 cup	200	66	24	5.4	2.8	0.07	0.07	0.2
VI	*Egg, milk and meat preparation*									
1.	Meat curry	1 serving	128	220	116	18	2.7	0.1	0.01	2.1
2.	Omelet	1 serving	39	77	5.8	5.7	0.5	0.03	0.1	1
3.	Meat fry	1 serving	142	339	21.8	26	4.5	0.23	0.2	3.3
4.	Fish fry	1 serving	100	220	16.2	16.2	1.4	0.05	0.45	1.2
5.	Rice, mutton pulao	2 servings	341	686	39	39	63.6	0.1	0.22	1.5
VII	*Preparation containing milk*									
1.	Coffee	1 cup	200	104	3.8	3.4	14.4	0.1	0.1	1.2
2.	Tea	1 cup	200	72	1.4	1.6	13	0.06	0.04	-
3.	Cocoa	1 cup	200	174	7.5	20.2	20.2	0.2	0.15	0.3
4.	Wheat payasam	1 cup	154	178	3.4	31.5	31.5	0.09	0.08	0.4
5.	Rice payasam	1 cup	266	227	3.7	44.3	44.3	0.14	0.1	4.7
6.	Rice porridge	1 cup	280	263	7.6	44.7	35.9	0.3	0.2	0.7
7.	Soy porridge	1 cup	154	178	7.7	44	44.7	0.07	0.14	0.4
8.	Wheat porridge	1 cup	280	263	7.6	44.7	35.9	0.3	0.22	0.7
9.	Ragi porridge	1 cup	193	317	8.7	52.7	35.9	0.24	0.22	1
10.	Milk (cow)	1 cup	200	130	7	9.8	52.7	0.12	0.1	0.4

Health education regarding importance of nutrition

Time	Goals/Objectives	Activities		Audiovisual (AV) aids	Method of teaching	Evaluation
		Teacher	Client			

Contd...

Contd...

Time	Goals/Objectives	Activities		Audiovisual (AV) aids	Method of teaching	Evaluation
		Teacher	Client			

Contd...

Contd...

Time	Goals/Objectives	Activities		Audiovisual (AV) aids	Method of teaching	Evaluation
		Teacher	Client			

Contd...

Contd...

Time	Goals/Objectives	Activities		Audiovisual (AV) aids	Method of teaching	Evaluation
		Teacher	Client			

Contd...

Contd...

Time	Goals/Objectives	Activities		Audiovisual (AV) aids	Method of teaching	Evaluation
		Teacher	Client			

Evaluation for Cooking Demonstration

Name of the student : ____________________

Batch (year) : ____________________

Name of the recipient : ____________________

Communication area : ____________________

Date and time : ____________________

Sl No.	Criteria	Marks allotted	Marks obtained
1.	Required item to be selected according to the needs of recipe	2	
2.	Prepared and summated on the time	2	
3.	Assessment of nutrition status of family	2	
4.	Family members interest	2	
5.	Way of preparation (hygiene, neat manner)	2	
6.	Selection of place and vessels	2	
7.	Way of serving	2	
8.	Cost benefit	2	
9.	Calculation of nutritive values for food items	2	
10.	Feedback from the family members	2	
	Total	**20**	

Signature of the Student
Date:

Signature of the Clinical Coordinator
Date:

Signature of the HOD of Community Health Nursing
Date:

Observation Visit

Case 1

Place of Visit : ____________________

Date of Visit : ____________________

Time : From: __________ To: __________

Name of the Institution : ____________________

Distance from the College : ____________________

Total Area : ____________________

Type of the Institution : ____________________

Head of the Institution : ____________________

Total Number of Employees of Working : ____________________

Name of the Organizer of the Student : ____________________

Introduction

General Objectives of the Visit

Organizational Chart

Philosophy of Organization

Aims and Objectives of Organization

Functions of Organization

Budgeting of Organization

Importance of Student Nurses

Summary

Conclusion

Signature of the Student
Date:

Signature of the Supervisor
Date:

Signature of the HOD of Community Health Nursing
Date:

Evaluation for Cooking Demonstration

Name of the student : ______________________________

Date and year : ______________________________

Place of visit : ______________________________

Sl No.	Criteria	Marks allotted	Marks obtained
1.	Introduction	2	
2.	Objectives of visit	3	
3.	Organizational setup	1	
4.	Functions of organization	3	
5.	Supportive agencies	2	
6.	Role of student nurses participation in the visit	3	
7.	Summary and conclusion	2	
8.	Budgeting of organization	2	
9.	Time management	2	
	Total	**20**	

Observation Visit

Case 2

Place of Visit : ____________________

Date of Visit : ____________________

Time : From: __________ To: __________

Name of the Institution : ____________________

Distance from the College : ____________________

Total Area : ____________________

Type of the Institution : ____________________

Head of the Institution : ____________________

Total Number of Employees of Working : ____________________

Name of the Organizer of the Student : ____________________

Introduction

General Objectives of the Visit

Organizational Chart

Philosophy of Organization

Aims and Objectives of Organization

Functions of Organization

Budgeting of Organization

Importance of Student Nurses

Summary

Conclusion

Signature of the Student
Date:

Signature of the Supervisor
Date:

Signature of the HOD of Community Health Nursing
Date:

Evaluation for Cooking Demonstration

Name of the student : ____________________

Date and year : ____________________

Place of visit : ____________________

Sl No.	Criteria	Marks allotted	Marks obtained
1.	Introduction	2	
2.	Objectives of visit	3	
3.	Organizational setup	1	
4.	Functions of organization	3	
5.	Supportive agencies	2	
6.	Role of student nurses participation in the visit	3	
7.	Summary and conclusion	2	
8.	Budgeting of organization	2	
9.	Time management	2	
	Total	**20**	

Observation Visit

Case 3

Place of Visit : ____________________

Date of Visit : ____________________

Time : From: ____________ To: ____________

Name of the Institution : ____________________

Distance from the College : ____________________

Total Area : ____________________

Type of the Institution : ____________________

Head of the Institution : ____________________

Total Number of Employees of Working : ____________________

Name of the Organizer of the Student : ____________________

Introduction

General Objectives of the Visit

Organizational Chart

Philosophy of Organization

Aims and Objectives of Organization

Functions of Organization

Budgeting of Organization

Importance of Student Nurses

Summary

Conclusion

Signature of the Student
Date:

Signature of the Supervisor
Date:

Signature of the HOD of Community Health Nursing
Date:

Evaluation for Cooking Demonstration

Name of the student : ________________

Date and year : ________________

Place of visit : ________________

Sl No.	Criteria	Marks allotted	Marks obtained
1.	Introduction	2	
2.	Objectives of visit	3	
3.	Organizational setup	1	
4.	Functions of organization	3	
5.	Supportive agencies	2	
6.	Role of student nurses participation in the visit	3	
7.	Summary and conclusion	2	
8.	Budgeting of organization	2	
9.	Time management	2	
	Total	**20**	

Observation Visit

Case 4

Place of Visit : ____________________

Date of Visit : ____________________

Time : From: ____________ To: ____________

Name of the Institution : ____________________

Distance from the College : ____________________

Total Area : ____________________

Type of the Institution : ____________________

Head of the Institution : ____________________

Total Number of Employees of Working : ____________________

Name of the Organizer of the Student : ____________________

Introduction

General Objectives of the Visit

Organizational Chart

Philosophy of Organization

Aims and Objectives of Organization

Functions of Organization

Budgeting of Organization

Importance of Student Nurses

Summary

Conclusion

Signature of the Student
Date:

Signature of the Supervisor
Date:

Signature of the HOD of Community Health Nursing
Date:

Evaluation for Cooking Demonstration

Name of the student : ________________

Date and year : ________________

Place of visit : ________________

Sl No.	Criteria	Marks allotted	Marks obtained
1.	Introduction	2	
2.	Objectives of visit	3	
3.	Organizational setup	1	
4.	Functions of organization	3	
5.	Supportive agencies	2	
6.	Role of student nurses participation in the visit	3	
7.	Summary and conclusion	2	
8.	Budgeting of organization	2	
9.	Time management	2	
	Total	**20**	

Bag Technique Procedure

Case 1

Name of the Student : ____________________

Name of the Procedure : ____________________

Date of the Procedure : ____________________

Name of the Patient : ____________________

House Number : ____________________

Age/Sex of the Patient : ____________________

Education of the Patient : ____________________

Occupation of the Patient : ____________________

Requirement of the Procedure : ____________________

Name of the Supervisor : ____________________

Nursing Diagnosis of the Patient

Objectives of the Procedure

Requirement of Articles

Initial Preparation of Patient

Procedure

Health Education about Procedure

Summary

Conclusion

Checklist for Bag Technique Procedure

Sl No.	Knowledge and skills	Grading	Score obtained by the student
1.	Essential supplies and equipment	2	
2.	Explain the procedure to the patient	2	
3.	Spreading of newspaper	2	
4.	Way of opening the bag	2	
5.	Handling of handwashing articles	2	
6.	Handwashing techniques	3	
7.	Handling necessary articles for the procedure	2	
8.	Maintain comfortable position of the patient	2	
9.	Maintain good communication skills and knowledge	2	
10.	Performing the procedure	4	
11.	Discharge the waste	2	
12.	Replacement of the articles	2	
13.	Folding the newspapers	2	
14.	Wash hands and close the bag	2	
15.	Knowledge about the usage of the bag	2	
16.	Record the result	1	
17.	Report to the clinical instructor (supervisor)	1	
	Total marks scored	35	

Signature of the Student
Date:

Signature of the Supervisor
Date:

Signature of the HOD of Community Health Nursing
Date:

Bag Technique Procedure
Case 2

Name of the Student : ______________________________

Name of the Procedure : ______________________________

Date of the Procedure : ______________________________

Name of the Patient : ______________________________

House Number : ______________________________

Age/Sex of the Patient : ______________________________

Education of the Patient : ______________________________

Occupation of the Patient : ______________________________

Requirement of the Procedure : ______________________________

Name of the Supervisor : ______________________________

Nursing Diagnosis of the Patient

Objectives of the Procedure

Requirement of Articles

Initial Preparation of Patient

Procedure

Health Education about Procedure

Summary

Conclusion

Checklist for Bag Technique Procedure

Sl No.	Knowledge and skills	Grading	Score obtained by the student
1.	Essential supplies and equipment	2	
2.	Explain the procedure to the patient	2	
3.	Spreading of newspaper	2	
4.	Way of opening the bag	2	
5.	Handling of handwashing articles	2	
6.	Handwashing techniques	3	
7.	Handling necessary articles for the procedure	2	
8.	Maintain comfortable position of the patient	2	
9.	Maintain good communication skills and knowledge	2	
10.	Performing the procedure	4	
11.	Discharge the waste	2	
12.	Replacement of the articles	2	
13.	Folding the newspapers	2	
14.	Wash hands and close the bag	2	
15.	Knowledge about the usage of the bag	2	
16.	Record the result	1	
17.	Report to the clinical instructor (supervisor)	1	
	Total marks scored	**35**	

Signature of the Student
Date:

Signature of the Supervisor
Date:

Signature of the HOD of Community Health Nursing
Date:

Bag Technique Procedure

Case 3

Name of the Student : ____________________

Name of the Procedure : ____________________

Date of the Procedure : ____________________

Name of the Patient : ____________________

House Number : ____________________

Age/Sex of the Patient : ____________________

Education of the Patient : ____________________

Occupation of the Patient : ____________________

Requirement of the Procedure : ____________________

Name of the Supervisor : ____________________

Nursing Diagnosis of the Patient

Objectives of the Procedure

Requirement of Articles

Initial Preparation of Patient

Procedure

Health Education about Procedure

Summary

Conclusion

Checklist for Bag Technique Procedure

Sl No.	Knowledge and skills	Grading	Score obtained by the student
1.	Essential supplies and equipment	2	
2.	Explain the procedure to the patient	2	
3.	Spreading of newspaper	2	
4.	Way of opening the bag	2	
5.	Handling of handwashing articles	2	
6.	Handwashing techniques	3	
7.	Handling necessary articles for the procedure	2	
8.	Maintain comfortable position of the patient	2	
9.	Maintain good communication skills and knowledge	2	
10.	Performing the procedure	4	
11.	Discharge the waste	2	
12.	Replacement of the articles	2	
13.	Folding the newspapers	2	
14.	Wash hands and close the bag	2	
15.	Knowledge about the usage of the bag	2	
16.	Record the result	1	
17.	Report to the clinical instructor (supervisor)	1	
	Total marks scored	35	

Signature of the Student
Date:

Signature of the Supervisor
Date:

Signature of the HOD of Community Health Nursing
Date:

Bag Technique Procedure

Case 4

Name of the Student : ______________________

Name of the Procedure : ______________________

Date of the Procedure : ______________________

Name of the Patient : ______________________

House Number : ______________________

Age/Sex of the Patient : ______________________

Education of the Patient : ______________________

Occupation of the Patient : ______________________

Requirement of the Procedure : ______________________

Name of the Supervisor : ______________________

Nursing Diagnosis of the Patient

Objectives of the Procedure

Requirement of Articles

Initial Preparation of Patient

Procedure

Health Education about Procedure

Summary

Conclusion

Checklist for Bag Technique Procedure

Sl No.	Knowledge and skills	Grading	Score obtained by the student
1.	Essential supplies and equipment	2	
2.	Explain the procedure to the patient	2	
3.	Spreading of newspaper	2	
4.	Way of opening the bag	2	
5.	Handling of handwashing articles	2	
6.	Handwashing techniques	3	
7.	Handling necessary articles for the procedure	2	
8.	Maintain comfortable position of the patient	2	
9.	Maintain good communication skills and knowledge	2	
10.	Performing the procedure	4	
11.	Discharge the waste	2	
12.	Replacement of the articles	2	
13.	Folding the newspapers	2	
14.	Wash hands and close the bag	2	
15.	Knowledge about the usage of the bag	2	
16.	Record the result	1	
17.	Report to the clinical instructor (supervisor)	1	
	Total marks scored	**35**	

Signature of the Student
Date:

Signature of the Supervisor
Date:

Signature of the HOD of Community Health Nursing
Date:

Bag Technique Procedure

Case 5

Name of the Student : ____________________

Name of the Procedure : ____________________

Date of the Procedure : ____________________

Name of the Patient : ____________________

House Number : ____________________

Age/Sex of the Patient : ____________________

Education of the Patient : ____________________

Occupation of the Patient : ____________________

Requirement of the Procedure : ____________________

Name of the Supervisor : ____________________

Nursing Diagnosis of the Patient

Objectives of the Procedure

Requirement of Articles

Initial Preparation of Patient

Procedure

Health Education about Procedure

Summary

Conclusion

Checklist for Bag Technique Procedure

Sl No.	Knowledge and skills	Grading	Score obtained by the student
1.	Essential supplies and equipment	2	
2.	Explain the procedure to the patient	2	
3.	Spreading of newspaper	2	
4.	Way of opening the bag	2	
5.	Handling of handwashing articles	2	
6.	Handwashing techniques	3	
7.	Handling necessary articles for the procedure	2	
8.	Maintain comfortable position of the patient	2	
9.	Maintain good communication skills and knowledge	2	
10.	Performing the procedure	4	
11.	Discharge the waste	2	
12.	Replacement of the articles	2	
13.	Folding the newspapers	2	
14.	Wash hands and close the bag	2	
15.	Knowledge about the usage of the bag	2	
16.	Record the result	1	
17.	Report to the clinical instructor (supervisor)	1	
	Total marks scored	**35**	

Signature of the Student
Date:

Signature of the Supervisor
Date:

Signature of the HOD of Community Health Nursing
Date:

Health Education

Case 1

Name of the Student : ____________________

Topic : ____________________

Method of Teaching : ____________________

Audiovisual Aids : ____________________

Duration : ____________________

Place : ____________________

Date : ____________________

Focus Group : ____________________

Needs of Education

Objectives of Education

Health education regarding importance of nutrition

Time	Goals/Objectives	Activities		Audiovisual (AV) aids	Method of teaching	Evaluation
		Teacher	Client			

Contd...

Contd...

Time	Goals/Objectives	Activities		Audiovisual (AV) aids	Method of teaching	Evaluation
		Teacher	Client			

Contd...

Contd...

Time	Goals/Objectives	Activities		Audiovisual (AV) aids	Method of teaching	Evaluation
		Teacher	Client			

Contd...

Contd...

Time	Goals/Objectives	Activities		Audiovisual (AV) aids	Method of teaching	Evaluation
		Teacher	Client			

Contd...

Contd...

Time	Goals/Objectives	Activities		Audiovisual (AV) aids	Method of teaching	Evaluation
		Teacher	Client			

Evaluation for Cooking Demonstration

Name of the student : ____________________

Date and time : ____________________

Topic : ____________________

Community area : ____________________

Name of the clinical instructor : ____________________

Sl No.	Criteria	Excellent	Very good	Average	Poor	Very poor
		5	4	3	2	1
1.	Content: a. Relevant b. Adequate c. Organization d. Depth of knowledge e. Recent advancement					
2.	Presentation: a. Voice audible b. Clarity c. Modulation d. Confidence e. Posture language f. Motivated g. Group participation h. Feedback					
3.	Audiovisual aids: a. Appropriate b. Preparation c. Visibility d. Proper usage e. Follow principles f. Replace of material g. Time management					
	Total					

Comments	

Signature of the Student
Date:

Signature of the HOD of Community Health Nursing
Date:

Health Education

Case 2

Name of the Student : ____________________

Topic : ____________________

Method of Teaching : ____________________

Audiovisual Aids : ____________________

Duration : ____________________

Place : ____________________

Date : ____________________

Focus Group : ____________________

Needs of Education

Objectives of Education

Health education regarding importance of nutrition

Time	Goals/Objectives	Activities		Audiovisual (AV) aids	Method of teaching	Evaluation
		Teacher	Client			

Contd...

Contd...

Time	Goals/Objectives	Activities		Audiovisual (AV) aids	Method of teaching	Evaluation
		Teacher	Client			

Contd...

Contd...

Time	Goals/Objectives	Activities		Audiovisual (AV) aids	Method of teaching	Evaluation
		Teacher	Client			

Contd...

Contd...

Time	Goals/Objectives	Activities		Audiovisual (AV) aids	Method of teaching	Evaluation
		Teacher	Client			

Contd...

Contd...

Time	Goals/Objectives	Activities		Audiovisual (AV) aids	Method of teaching	Evaluation
		Teacher	Client			

Evaluation for Cooking Demonstration

Name of the student : ________________________

Date and time : ________________________

Topic : ________________________

Community area : ________________________

Name of the clinical instructor : ________________________

Sl No.	Criteria	Excellent	Very good	Average	Poor	Very poor
		5	4	3	2	1
1.	Content: a. Relevant b. Adequate c. Organization d. Depth of knowledge e. Recent advancement					
2.	Presentation: a. Voice audible b. Clarity c. Modulation d. Confidence e. Posture language f. Motivated g. Group participation h. Feedback					
3.	Audiovisual aids: a. Appropriate b. Preparation c. Visibility d. Proper usage e. Follow principles f. Replace of material g. Time management					
	Total					

Comments	

Signature of the Student
Date:

Signature of the HOD of Community Health Nursing
Date:

Audiovisual Aids Preparation

Case 1

Charts

Introduction

Objectives

Principles

Method of Preparation

Conclusion

Diorama

Introduction

Objectives

Principles

Method of Preparation

Conclusion

Flannelgraphs

Introduction

Objectives

Principles

Method of Preparation

Conclusion

Flash Card

Introduction

Objectives

Principles

Method of Preparation

Conclusion

Flip Chart

Introduction

Objectives

Principles

Method of Preparation

Conclusion

Pamphlet (or) Leaflet

Introduction

Objectives

Principles

Method of Preparation

Conclusion

Poster

Introduction

Objectives

Principles

Method of Preparation

Conclusion

Audiovisual Aids Preparation

Case 2

Charts

Introduction

Objectives

Principles

Method of Preparation

Conclusion

Diorama

Introduction

Objectives

Principles

Method of Preparation

Conclusion

Flannelgraphs

Introduction

Objectives

Principles

Method of Preparation

Conclusion

Flash Card

Introduction

Objectives

Principles

Method of Preparation

Conclusion

Flip Chart

Introduction

Objectives

Principles

Method of Preparation

Conclusion

Pamphlet (or) Leaflet

Introduction

Objectives

Principles

Method of Preparation

Conclusion

Poster

Introduction

Objectives

Principles

Method of Preparation

Conclusion

Audiovisual Aids Preparation

Case 3

Charts

Introduction

Objectives

Principles

Method of Preparation

Conclusion

Diorama

Introduction

Objectives

Principles

Method of Preparation

Conclusion

Flannelgraphs

Introduction

Objectives

Principles

Method of Preparation

Conclusion

Flash Card

Introduction

Objectives

Principles

Method of Preparation

Conclusion

Flip Chart

Introduction

Objectives

Principles

Method of Preparation

Conclusion

Pamphlet (or) Leaflet

Introduction

Objectives

Principles

Method of Preparation

Conclusion

Poster

Introduction

Objectives

Principles

Method of Preparation

Conclusion

Audiovisual Aids Preparation

Case 4

Charts

Introduction

Objectives

Principles

Method of Preparation

Conclusion

Diorama

Introduction

Objectives

Principles

Method of Preparation

Conclusion

Flannelgraphs

Introduction

Objectives

Principles

Method of Preparation

Conclusion

Flash Card

Introduction

Objectives

Principles

Method of Preparation

Conclusion

Flip Chart

Introduction

Objectives

Principles

Method of Preparation

Conclusion

Pamphlet (or) Leaflet

Introduction

Objectives

Principles

Method of Preparation

Conclusion

Poster

Introduction

Objectives

Principles

Method of Preparation

Conclusion

Audiovisual Aids Preparation

Case 5

Charts

Introduction

Objectives

Principles

Method of Preparation

Conclusion

Diorama

Introduction

Objectives

Principles

Method of Preparation

Conclusion

Flannelgraphs

Introduction

Objectives

Principles

Method of Preparation

Conclusion

Flash Card

Introduction

Objectives

Principles

Method of Preparation

Conclusion

Flip Chart

Introduction

Objectives

Principles

Method of Preparation

Conclusion

Pamphlet (or) Leaflet

Introduction

Objectives

Principles

Method of Preparation

Conclusion

Poster

Introduction

Objectives

Principles

Method of Preparation

Conclusion

Audiovisual Aids Preparation

Case 6

Charts

Introduction

Objectives

Principles

Method of Preparation

Conclusion

Diorama

Introduction

Objectives

Principles

Method of Preparation

Conclusion

Flannelgraphs

Introduction

Objectives

Principles

Method of Preparation

Conclusion

Flash Card

Introduction

Objectives

Principles

Method of Preparation

Conclusion

Flip Chart

Introduction

Objectives

Principles

Method of Preparation

Conclusion

Pamphlet (or) Leaflet

Introduction

Objectives

Principles

Method of Preparation

Conclusion

Poster

Introduction

Objectives

Principles

Method of Preparation

Conclusion

Audiovisual Aids Preparation

Case 7

Charts

Introduction

Objectives

Principles

Method of Preparation

Conclusion

Diorama

Introduction

Objectives

Principles

Method of Preparation

Conclusion

Flannelgraphs

Introduction

Objectives

Principles

Method of Preparation

Conclusion

Flash Card

Introduction

Objectives

Principles

Method of Preparation

Conclusion

Flip Chart

Introduction

Objectives

Principles

Method of Preparation

Conclusion

Pamphlet (or) Leaflet

Introduction

Objectives

Principles

Method of Preparation

Conclusion

Poster

Introduction

Objectives

Principles

Method of Preparation

Conclusion

Organization of Health Camp

Introduction

Objectives of Health Camp

Need Assessment

Community Resource Organization

Identification of Needs and Problem

Discussion Based on Need and Problem to Identify with Influence People from the Community

Participatory Appraisal

Organizing the Resource (Doctors, Funding Resource, Physical Resource, Supplies and Articles, Manpower)

Evaluation Regarding Health Camp

Feedback from Community People